DENTAL ASSISTANT

775
Questions & Answers

Emily Andujo, RDH, BS, MS
Dental Hygiene Education
Pima Community College
Tucson, Arizona

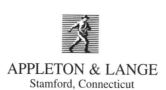

APPLETON & LANGE
Stamford, Connecticut

Copyright © 1998 by Appleton & Lange
A Simon & Schuster Company

www.appletonlange.com

98 99 00 01 02 / 10 9 8 7 6 5 4 3 2

Prentice Hall International (UK) Limited, *London*
Prentice Hall of Australia Pty. Limited, *Sydney*
Prentice Hall Canada. Inc., *Toronto*
Prentice Hall Hispanoamericana, S.A., *Mexico*
Prentice Hall of India Private Limited, *New Delhi*
Prentice Hall of Japan, Inc., *Tokyo*
Simon & Schuster Asia Pte. Ltd., *Singapore*
Editora Prentice Hall do Brasil Ltda., *Rio de Janeiro*
Prentice Hall, *Upper Saddle River, New Jersey*

Library of Congress Cataloging-in-Publication Data
Andujo, Emily.
    Dental assistant : 775 questions and answers / Emily
Andujo — 1st ed.
        p.   cm. — (Appleton & Lange's quick review)
    ISBN 0-8385-1526-6 (pbk. : alk. paper)
    1. Dental assistants—Examinations, questions, etc.   2. Dentistry—
Examinations, questions, etc. I. Title. II. Series: A&L's quick review.
    [DNLM: 1. Dental Care—examination questions.
    2. Dental Assistants—examination questions.   WU 18.2 A577d 1998]
RK60.5.A53   1998
617.6'0233'076—dc21
DNLM/DLC
for Library of Congress   97-30650

ISBN 0-8385-1526-6

Acquisitions Editor: Marinita Timban
Production Service: Inkwell Publishing Services
Production Editor: Lisa M. Guidone
Designer: Mary Skudlarek

PRINTED IN THE UNITED STATES OF AMERICA

Contents

Preface

Appleton & Lange's Quick Review: Dental Assistant is designed to act as a study companion for students who are (1) preparing for national board examinations and/or (2) pursuing self-assessment in dental assisting. This book enables the reader to review relevant material while becoming familiar with the types of questions given on board examinations.

A&L's Quick Review is divided into **six simulated examinations** with answers and explanations. A list of references for each question and answer is in the bibliography as additional review resources.

The practice tests focus on the content material outlined in the Dental Assisting National Board (DANB) task analysis guide. The certification examinations are composed of four different question formats: one best answer–single item, complex multiple choice or K-type, negative format, and matching. Each of the six practice tests has been designed according to this question format.

A comprehensive simulated exam is also provided to ensure that the test applicant has reviewed all of the content areas. Many of the DANB certification examinations overlap into other subject areas. For example, the practice tests on radiology and infection control include content that appears on the specialty examinations. Likewise, content in radiology and infection control appears in the General Chairside component of the DANB examination.

The DANB administers the board examinations electronically. Therefore, a study disk is included to help prepare you for this computerized format. The review program includes the following key features:

- Assessment of strengths and weaknesses
- Ability to create multiple customized practice tests
- Scoring and timer functions

Additional examination preparation material is provided in the companion book, *Dental Assistant Program Review and Exam Preparation (PREP)*. *PREP* provides a comprehensive overview of high-impact topics in dental assisting. Both books offer a thorough review for the certification examinations administered by the DANB.

We wish you luck on your certification examinations. We believe that you will find the questions, explanations, and format of the text to be of great assistance to you during your review.

Acknowledgments

I would like to thank Marinita Timban, Review Book Editor at Appleton & Lange, for her continued support and commitment to the integration of technology for *A&L's Quick Review Series* test preparation books. I would also like to acknowledge Lisa Guidone, Production Editor at Appleton & Lange, who provided guidance and support during the development of this book.

I would also like to thank the Dental Assisting Education Class of 1997 at Pima Community College for their suggestions and Pam Kercheval, CDA, Dental Assisting instructor.

I would like to thank my friends, colleagues, and contributors for their suggestions and encouragement. In particular to Olivia Ordonez, CDA, Dental Office Manager & Safety Coordinator, for her assistance and contribution to the chapter on Occupational Safety and to Lori Gagliardi, RDA, RDH, for her input on the content.

A special note of thanks to my computer mentor and soul mate for the extra patience displayed and the countless hours spent formatting, inputting, and editing this project to final perfection for copy. Thanks, "D."

Practice Test Questions 1: Chairside Assisting

DIRECTIONS (Questions 1–100): Each of the questions or incomplete statements in this section is followed by four suggested answers or completions. Select the **ONE** lettered answer or completion that is **BEST** in each case.

1. Before rendering any type of dental treatment on a patient, the dental assistant must
   A. obtain a complete medical history
   B. explain the office policy on broken appointments
   C. approve the patient's dental insurance
   D. obtain a complete set of radiographs

2. The main role of the assistant in preventive dentistry is
   A. dispensing fluoride rinses
   B. taking x-rays
   C. patient education
   D. recording vital signs

3. Before applying a topical fluoride gel to the teeth the assistant must
   A. set up a recall appointment
   B. dry the teeth thoroughly
   C. review the x-rays
   D. provide plaque control instructions

4. Teeth most likely to benefit from the application of pit and fissure sealants are
   A. anterior teeth only
   B. posterior teeth with small carious occlusal pits
   C. partially erupted first permanent molars
   D. posterior teeth with deep pits and fissures

5. The assistant's eye level when seated is
   A. even with that of the dentist
   B. 4″ to 6″ below that of the dentist
   C. 4″ to 6″ above the patient's shoulder
   D. 4″ to 6″ above that of the dentist

6. If a right-handed operator is preparing a mandibular right molar for a crown preparation, the assistant retracts
   A. the tongue
   B. the cheek
   C. both the tongue and the cheek
   D. neither the tongue nor the cheek

7. Protective barriers are necessary when
   A. confirming appointments
   B. presenting toothbrush instruction
   C. ordering supplies
   D. sterilizing instruments

8. The dental assistant observes the patient during the assessment phase of evaluation for all of the following **EXCEPT**
   A. anxiety level of patient
   B. patient's insurance coverage
   C. signs of substance (drug) abuse
   D. signs of physical abuse

9. When working in the anterior part of the mouth, the high-volume evacuation tip is held
   A. below the incisal edge of the tooth being prepared
   B. on the opposite side of the tooth being prepared
   C. in the retromolar area
   D. in the vestibule

10. Angle's classification of malocclusion is based on the
    A. shape of the maxilla
    B. relationship between the first molars and the orbit of the eye
    C. relationship between the maxillary and mandibular first molars
    D. number of teeth in the mandible

11. A normal blood pressure reading is
    A. 120/80
    B. 140/100
    C. 160/80
    D. 180/60

12. During the administration of local anesthesia, aspiration will
    A. damage the mandibular artery
    B. be extremely painful
    C. determine if the lumen of the needle is in a blood vessel
    D. ensure profound anesthesia

13. The condition in which a patient lacks oxygen is called
    A. hyperventilation
    B. hypoxia
    C. anoxia
    D. syncope

14. The patient's clinical record must include
    A. laboratory invoices
    B. medical health questionnaire
    C. study models
    D. insurance forms

15. The assistant holds the hand instrument to be transferred between the
    A. thumb and forefinger
    B. small finger and palm
    C. thumb and palm
    D. small finger and forefinger

16. The fulcrum digit used in the modified pen grasp is the
    A. thumb
    B. index finger
    C. middle finger
    D. ring finger

17. If caries is present on the lingual pit of tooth No. 7, it is classified as
    A. Class V
    B. Class IV
    C. Class I
    D. Class III

18. The purpose of relining a denture is to
    A. alter the occlusion
    B. fill in the voids of the denture base for better readaptation
    C. make a custom-made tray
    D. take a bite registration

19. The matrix band should be removed
    A. firmly with a hemostat
    B. quickly with a sliding motion
    C. slowly in an occlusal direction
    D. quickly through the contact area

20. The color of the nitrous oxide cylinder tank is always
    A. blue
    B. green
    C. yellow
    D. red

21. A patient who jumps out of the chair after being treated in the supine position may experience
    A. signs of giddiness
    B. xerostomia
    C. signs of syncope
    D. increase in systolic pressure

22. When loading a tray with irreversible hydrocolloid
   A. more material is placed posteriorly
   B. more material is placed anteriorly
   C. more material is placed in the palatal area
   D. the material is placed evenly in the entire tray

23. A mesial occlusal cavity preparation is an example of a
   A. Class I cavity preparation
   B. Class II cavity preparation
   C. Class III cavity preparation
   D. Class IV cavity preparation

24. During the placement of a rubber dam, a blunt instrument can be used to
   A. ligate the rubber dam
   B. invert the rubber dam
   C. punch small holes for the anterior teeth in the rubber dam
   D. secure the clamp

25. The rubber dam napkin is used to
   A. place the dam
   B. secure the dam
   C. avoid irritation around the patient's face
   D. help the patient swallow

26. A lubricant can be used on the rubber dam to
   A. retard the flow of saliva
   B. help clamp the last tooth
   C. repair a torn dam
   D. make it easier for the dam to be slipped between the teeth

27. A cavity preparation that includes the mesial incisal angle of a maxillary central incisor is classified as a
   A. Class I cavity preparation
   B. Class II cavity preparation
   C. Class III cavity preparation
   D. Class IV cavity preparation

28. Debridement of the cavity preparation refers to
   A. resisting dislodgement of filling materials
   B. retaining of filling material in the cavity preparation
   C. removal of debris from the cavity preparation
   D. removal of undermined enamel

29. Impression waxes are used
   A. for bite registration
   B. for study models
   C. to cast restorations
   D. to hold dies in position

30. During a Class II amalgam procedure, the rubber dam is removed
   A. before checking the patient's occlusion
   B. before condensing the amalgam
   C. before removing the matrix band
   D. after the matrix band is in position

31. Which of the following is **NOT** used to evaluate an amalgam restoration?
   A. Mirror
   B. Burnisher
   C. Articulating paper
   D. Dental floss

32. In application of the rubber dam, which tooth should be used as the anchor tooth?
   A. The tooth being prepared
   B. The most anterior tooth in the quadrant
   C. 1 or 2 teeth distal to the tooth being prepared
   D. 1 or 2 teeth mesial to the tooth being prepared

33. Removal of the rubber dam is accomplished by
   A. cutting the septal dam before removal
   B. stretching the dam for interproximal removal
   C. a quick snap
   D. stretching the dam with rubber dam forceps

34. Which of the following pieces of equipment should be disinfected after treatment of each patient?
   A. Handpieces
   B. Curettes
   C. Film holders
   D. Light handles

35. The purpose of palpating the neck of a patient is
   A. to determine TMJ dysfunction
   B. to feel enlarged lymph nodes
   C. to determine the size of extraoral x-ray film
   D. to make the patient feel more relaxed

36. In a mouth with poor oral hygiene, the white deposit that collects around the gingival margin of the teeth is
   A. dental plaque
   B. stain
   C. calculus
   D. leukoplakia

37. Coronal polishing of the occlusal surfaces is best accomplished with a
   A. prophy brush
   B. rubber cup
   C. porte polisher
   D. toothbrush

38. Instruments used on a patient with a history of hepatitis B should be sterilized by
   A. scrubbing with alcohol
   B. placing in a dry oven for 20 min.
   C. a cold disinfectant method
   D. a steam sterilization (autoclave) method

39. A good method of keeping a mouth mirror from fogging is
   A. hold it in cold water
   B. sponge it with alcohol
   C. blast it with cool air
   D. rub mirror against patient's buccal mucosa

40. A cavity varnish is applied to the
    A. enamel walls only
    B. dentinal tubules only
    C. walls and floor of a cavity preparation
    D. floor of the cavity preparation only

41. Calcium hydroxide is used because it
    A. seals the dentinal tubules
    B. acts as a thermal insulator under metallic restoration
    C. reduces marginal leakage around the restoration
    D. stimulates the formation of secondary dentin

42. When taking an alginate impression of the upper arch the patient should be seated in a (an)
    A. slightly reclined position with the chin tilted downward
    B. upright position with head tilted forward
    C. upright position with head tilted back
    D. supine position

43. To ensure that the set alginate impression remains firmly attached in the tray during removal from the mouth, which tray is used?
    A. Water-cooled perforated tray
    B. Perforated plastic or Rim-lock tray
    C. Custom-made compound tray
    D. Styrofoam disposable tray

44. The reason for using a plastic spatula when mixing a composite resin is that the
    A. material sticks more readily to metal
    B. cold metal would adversely affect the setting time of the material
    C. material would become discolored with a metal spatula
    D. plastic spatulas are disposable

45. Which of the following statements is true concerning placement of a wedge for a matrix?
    A. It should separate the teeth slightly
    B. It should be placed only when a rubber dam is used
    C. It should be placed so that one edge extends below the gingiva
    D. It should be placed in the smallest embrasure

46. What type of matrix band is required for molars having deep gingival preparations?
  A. Universal metal matrix bands
  B. Mylar strips
  C. Wide gingival extension metal molar bands
  D. Class V contour matrix bands

47. A Tofflemire matrix prepared for tooth No. 28 also can be used on teeth in which other quadrant?
  A. Maxillary left
  B. Mandibular right
  C. Maxillary right
  D. Mandibular left

48. The best way to prevent gagging during impression taking is to
  A. use cold water when mixing the alginate
  B. instruct patient to breathe through their nose and not through their mouth
  C. fill the tray as much as possible
  D. take the upper arch impression first

49. The use of outdated films, stray radiation, or unsafe darkroom light would most likely cause a
  A. blurred film
  B. very light film
  C. clear film
  D. fogged film

50. A radiation detection badge is essential for use in the dental office to
  A. protect the x-ray machine from damage caused by overheating
  B. estimate the radiation absorbed by the wearer
  C. reduce the exposure of the patient to radiation
  D. identify the operator as a licensed x-ray technician

51. Before application of a topical anesthetic, the area should be
  A. rinsed with water
  B. wiped with an alcohol sponge
  C. dried with a 2×2 gauze
  D. completely numb

52. A temporary filling is best packed with
   A. heavy pressure
   B. a condenser
   C. a moist cotton pellet
   D. a ball burnisher

53. What instruments are best suited for removing excess cement from the teeth?
   A. Spatula and scalpel
   B. A dull chisel and mallet
   C. Ball burnisher and explorer
   D. Explorer and scaler

54. When working with a visible light cure unit
   A. the dental unit light must be set on low
   B. a face shield may be worn in place of a face mask
   C. protective visible light eyewear is required
   D. protective eyewear is not necessary

55. When placing a temporary filling, it is **NOT** important to
   A. carve detailed anatomy
   B. seal the margins completely
   C. make sure it is in proper occlusion
   D. contact the adjacent tooth

56. The primary use of a matrix band is to
   A. stabilize the tooth
   B. provide the missing wall in a proximal surface cavity
   C. aid in restoring the anatomy to a Class I restoration
   D. restore more than one tooth at a time in the same quadrant

57. A properly placed Tofflemire matrix band should be
   A. mounted with the retainer on the lingual side of the arch
   B. at least 3 mm above the occlusal and 3 mm below the gingival attachment
   C. at least 2 mm above the occlusal margin and 1 mm below the gingival margin of the preparation
   D. mounted with the retainer on the buccal side of the maxillary arch and on the lingual side of the mandibular arch

58. Dental stone is used
  A. to pour all irreversible hydrocolloid impressions
  B. for occlusal registration
  C. to construct casts used in denture construction
  D. when plaster is not available

59. Which of the following is **NOT** a hand cutting instrument?
  A. Spoon excavator
  B. Hoe
  C. Gingival margin trimmer
  D. Beavertail burnisher

60. When using a Tofflemire matrix retainer, the diagonal slot should face
  A. toward the occlusal surface
  B. toward the lingual surface
  C. toward the incisal edge
  D. toward the gingiva

61. Flour of pumice should be moist when used to polish tooth surfaces because
  A. wet agents abrade faster than dry agents
  B. wet agents are more abrasive than dry agents
  C. wet agents cause less frictional heat than do dry agents
  D. wetting causes alteration of particle size

62. Light pressure should be used when polishing with a rubber cup so as not to cause the cup to
  A. flange into the gingival sulcus
  B. fray
  C. unscrew from the prophy angle
  D. cause any unnecessary frictional heat

63. An example of an extrinsic stain is
  A. blackline stain
  B. tetracycline stain
  C. hypoplasia stain
  D. silver nitrate stain

64. Tin oxide may be used as a polishing agent for
  A. acrylic restorations
  B. metallic restorations
  C. porcelain crowns
  D. ortho appliances

65. Bleaching procedures are performed when
  A. polishing of the teeth cannot be performed
  B. extrinsic stains exist
  C. artificial teeth have become stained
  D. intrinsic stains exist

66. Tying dental floss around the rubber dam clamp
  A. ligates it more securely to the tooth
  B. keeps the rubber dam in place
  C. prevents accidental swallowing of the clamp
  D. is never done

67. When seating the rubber dam clamp
  A. the lingual jaws are placed first
  B. the buccal jaws are placed first
  C. both are placed at the same time
  D. it makes no difference which are placed first

68. The most common form of fluoride used with the rigid tray system is
  A. sodium fluoride (NaF)
  B. stannous fluoride paste
  C. liquid fluoride supplements
  D. acidulated phosphate fluoride gel

69. Before pulp testing the teeth with a vitalometer, the teeth must be
  A. polished
  B. dried
  C. moistened
  D. flossed

70. A very low reading on the vitalometer (1–2) probably indicates
  A. hyperemia
  B. necrotic pulp
  C. dead pulp
  D. normal pulp

71. When testing the pulp of a tooth with an electric pulp tester, a high reading (9–10) indicates that the tooth is
    A. hyperemic
    B. near death
    C. nonvital
    D. normal

72. Before placing an x-ray film in the patient's mouth, the assistant must perform all of the following **EXCEPT**
    A. place a lead apron on the patient
    B. remove any appliances from the patient's mouth
    C. perform preliminary oral inspection
    D. chart existing restorations

73. Obtaining a measurement of the length of the root canal ensures
    A. profound anesthesia
    B. not irritating the periapical tissues by extending instruments beyond the apex of the root
    C. a sterile root canal
    D. no future pain

74. Endodontic files are used
    A. to enlarge the root canal
    B. to remove the contents of the pulp chamber
    C. as drains in an endodontic abscess
    D. to reduce the occlusal forces on an endodontically treated tooth

75. Gutta-percha is used to
    A. irrigate the root canal
    B. gain access to the root canal
    C. fill the root canal
    D. sterilize the root canal

76. A dilute sodium hypochlorite solution is recommended for cleaning
    A. partial dentures with metal clasps
    B. full dentures
    C. orthodontic bands
    D. mouths with heavy plaque accumulation

77. The Dental Practice Act
    A. is operated as an agency of the federal government
    B. is under the jurisdiction of the American Dental Association
    C. defines the practice of and regulates dentistry in each state
    D. certifies dental assistants

78. Removal of the coronal portion of the pulp is called
    A. pulp capping
    B. pulpotomy
    C. apical retention
    D. indirect pulp capping

79. Full coverage of a deciduous molar usually indicates the use of
    A. an amalgam crown
    B. an acrylic crown
    C. a stainless steel crown
    D. a porcelain crown

80. An apicoectomy is the
    A. chemical sterilization of the root apex
    B. root canal treatment of primary teeth
    C. procedure performed before reinforcing an endodontically treated tooth
    D. surgical removal of the apex of the root

81. Hemisection refers to
    A. an irreversible pulpitis
    B. a desensitizing solution
    C. the removal of a root from a multirooted tooth
    D. the removal of the root apex

82. A postextraction dressing can be used
    A. on all surgical sites
    B. only after third molar extractions
    C. when blood begins to ooze from the alveolus
    D. when there is loss of the blood clot in an extraction site

83. After an extraction, the best technique to stop bleeding is
    A. medicating with antibiotics
    B. applying indirect pressure

    C. applying direct pressure

    D. placing a drain in the extraction socket

84. Rinsing with warm salt water

    A. causes clot formation

    B. helps relieve pain

    C. causes edema

    D. decreases the number of oral microbes

85. The suture material that can be resorbed by the body is

    A. gut

    B. nylon

    C. white silk

    D. black silk

86. Postextraction dressings are removed and changed

    A. when the sutures are removed

    B. every 1 to 2 days as needed

    C. once a week

    D. after clot formation

87. When removing sutures, you must cut

    A. anywhere, as long as you can get the suture out

    B. in back of the knot and pull knot through tissue

    C. just below the knot with suture scissors

    D. the knot off, then remove suture gently with a hemostat

88. In treatment of a dry socket, first irrigate the alveolus with

    A. alcohol

    B. cold water

    C. fluoride mouth rinse

    D. warm saline solution

89. When placing a periodontal dressing, it is necessary to

    A. ligate with dental tape for stability

    B. festoon the surface of the dressing for aesthetics

    C. allow sutures to be exposed

    D. extend a large bulk of material well into the vestibule for strength

90. Instructions after periodontal surgery should include all of the following **EXCEPT**
   A. no smoking
   B. no spicy or hot foods
   C. use of a disclosing agent
   D. high protein diet

91. The method used to remove periodontal dressings is
   A. use beaks of cotton pliers to catch edges and use a teasing motion
   B. use fingernail to catch edge of dressing and remove
   C. with cotton pliers forcibly pull material away from tissue
   D. use an ultrasonic scaler

92. Preparation of an anesthetic syringe by the assistant includes all of the following **EXCEPT**
   A. engaging the stylet
   B. placing the anesthetic in the carpule
   C. placement of the carpule in the syringe
   D. loosening the cap covering the needle

93. Incision and drainage are used to treat a
   A. periodontal abscess
   B. granuloma
   C. cyst
   D. furcation

94. Nitrous oxide is classified as a (an)
   A. local anesthetic
   B. analgesic
   C. barbiturate
   D. narcotic

95. Which of the following is a description of a patient receiving the proper level of nitrous oxide?
   A. Dilated pupils, high blood pressure
   B. Excitement, muscles relaxed
   C. Unconscious, respiration slow, blood pressure elevated
   D. Muscles relaxed, pupils normal, blood pressure lowered

96. Before administering nitrous oxide to the patient
   A. instruct patient to breathe through mouth
   B. give oxygen for 2 min.
   C. administer anesthesia
   D. apply a rubber dam

97. Which does **NOT** apply to nitrous oxide sedation?
   A. Instruct patient to hold breath for 30 sec., then inhale deeply
   B. Instruct patient to breathe through the nose
   C. Reassure patient and project positive thoughts
   D. Never leave the room while patient is under nitrous oxide sedation

98. What is the treatment when a patient reaches the excitement stage of nitrous oxide sedation?
   A. No treatment necessary
   B. Give more anesthesia or wait until the drug wears off
   C. Decrease nitrous flow
   D. Increase nitrous flow

99. On the nitrous oxide unit, the flowmeter
   A. indicates the pressure of gas within the cylinder
   B. controls the breathing bag gas reservoir flow
   C. provides the operator with a guide to the volume of gas flowing to the patient
   D. transports gas from unit to mask

100. When working with nitrous oxide, all of the following apply **EXCEPT**
   A. monitor vital signs before administration
   B. work in a well-ventilated room
   C. nosepiece must be sterilized
   D. assistant may administer nitrous oxide if requested by patient

---

DIRECTIONS (Questions 101–113): For each of the items in this section, **ONE** or **MORE** of the numbered options is correct. Choose answer
  A. if only 1, 2, and 3 are correct
  B. if only 1 and 3 are correct
  C. if only 2 and 4 are correct
  D. if only 4 is correct
  E. if all are correct

---

101. Study models are used
  1. as references in orthodontic cases
  2. to show shape, size, and position of teeth
  3. as an aid in treatment planning
  4. to fabricate night guards

102. The rubber cup prophylaxis is indicated before placement of the rubber dam to
  1. polish the anterior restorations
  2. polish the posterior restorations
  3. remove the calculus
  4. avoid displacement of debris under the gingiva

103. Plaque control programs should contain
  1. oral physiotherapy instructions
  2. nutritional counseling
  3. behavioral modification techniques
  4. clinical examinations

104. When trimming study model casts with a model trimmer, it is best to
  1. wear protective glasses or a face shield
  2. begin with the mandibular cast
  3. allow sufficient water to flow through the model trimmer
  4. periodically check casts in an occluded position

105. Using a mouth mirror during an oral examination, the dental assistant may chart
  1. obvious lesions
  2. existing restorations
  3. missing teeth
  4. periodontal pockets

106. Functions of a good recall system may include
    1. provide reinforcement of good dental habits and correct any bad dental habits
    2. a prophy and fluoride treatment
    3. examination and evaluation by the dentist
    4. diagnosis of x-rays by the auxiliary

107. The mouth mirror may be used to
    1. retract the cheeks
    2. retract the tongue
    3. reflect light
    4. provide indirect vision

108. Wearing gloves can aid in preventing the contraction of
    1. epilepsy
    2. angina
    3. subacute bacterial endocarditis
    4. hepatitis

109. When cementing temporary crowns
    1. the amount of cement placed in the temporary crown depends on the type of crown
    2. a thick mix of cement is used so the bond is stronger
    3. the occlusion is checked after cementation and then adjusted
    4. it is not necessary to remove excess cement interproximally because it helps to maintain good contact

110. When applying pit and fissure sealants, it is best to
    1. use zinc phosphate cement
    2. use protective eyewear
    3. test occlusion and contacts
    4. apply a rubber dam

111. Glass ionomer cements may be used for
    1. permanent restorations
    2. luting procedures
    3. insulating bases
    4. sealants

112. When teaching toothbrushing, the important emphasis should be on
   1. brushing at least once a day
   2. brushing three times a day
   3. brushing before bedtime
   4. complete removal of plaque regardless of brushing time

113. Hand cutting instruments are used in restorative dentistry to
   1. remove deep carious lesions
   2. refine cavity preparations
   3. trim excess restorative material
   4. invaginate a rubber dam

DIRECTIONS (Questions 114–150): Each of the questions or incomplete statements in this section is followed by four suggested answers or completions. Select the **ONE** lettered answer or completion that is **BEST** in each case.

---

114. A mixed dentition consists of
   A. deciduous and permanent teeth existing simultaneously in a child's mouth
   B. deciduous teeth in the wrong places
   C. permanent teeth that are rotated
   D. permanent teeth in the wrong places

115. After topical fluoride application, patients should be instructed not to eat, drink, rinse, or brush their teeth for
   A. 5 min.
   B. 10 min.
   C. 30 min.
   D. 1 hr.

116. What appliances are used to maintain the space of a prematurely lost second primary molar?
   A. A space opener
   B. A space maintainer
   C. A space saver
   D. It is not necessary to maintain this space

117. Which technique for drying a cavity preparation can be injurious to the pulp?
   A. Cotton pledgets
   B. Short blasts of air
   C. A steady stream of air
   D. Use of 2×2 gauze

118. A supply company informs the office that an item that has been ordered is not available and will be shipped when it arrives. This is known as
   A. a back order
   B. an extra supply
   C. deficit spending
   D. a credit

119. Radiation exposure time for an edentulous patient should be
   A. increased by 25%
   B. the same as for a dentulous patient
   C. reduced by 25%
   D. reduced by 50%

120. What part of the partial denture holds it to the abutment tooth?
   A. The saddle area
   B. The rigid connector
   C. The surveyor
   D. The clasp

121. The part of the partial denture that lies over the ridge is called the
   A. saddle
   B. rigid connector
   C. surveyor
   D. clasp

122. The function of the preliminary impression in full denture construction is to
   A. construct wax rims
   B. help mount final casts
   C. construct a custom-made tray
   D. help make adjustments after insertion

123. A facebow is used to
  A. insert the denture in the patient's mouth
  B. contour the wax rims
  C. mount the upper cast on an articulator
  D. check the bite

124. Wax bite blocks are used to
  A. record vertical dimension
  B. determine sore spots
  C. construct custom-made trays
  D. flask dentures

125. What portion of the denture should **NOT** be polished?
  A. The part touching the tongue
  B. The part contacting the denture-bearing mucosa
  C. The part touching the cheeks
  D. All parts must be polished

126. To replace an intact tooth broken from a denture
  A. the site on the denture is roughened, some quick-cure acrylic is added, and the tooth is reset
  B. the tooth is luted to the denture with sticky wax
  C. the tooth is bonded back into place
  D. a new denture must be made

127. Heavy- and light-bodied impression materials are used with
  A. waxes
  B. alginate
  C. compound
  D. polysulfide (rubber base)

128. An immediate denture
  A. is constructed in one visit
  B. is made of shellac
  C. replaces only the anterior teeth
  D. is inserted during the same appointment in which the remaining teeth are extracted

129. Tissue conditioning
  - **A.** is used to help final casts
  - **B.** takes place at the time the denture is inserted in the patient's mouth
  - **C.** returns unhealthy tissue under a denture to a healthy state
  - **D.** is accomplished by using wax rims

130. Shade selection is accomplished using
  - **A.** natural light
  - **B.** the dental light
  - **C.** fluorescent light
  - **D.** black light

131. A function of a fixed bridge is
  - **A.** to help move teeth
  - **B.** to prevent movement of teeth
  - **C.** to make cleaning easier
  - **D.** to improve speech

132. The teeth that support a fixed bridge are called (refer to Fig. 1–1)
  - **A.** abutments
  - **B.** pontics
  - **C.** ridge laps
  - **D.** partials

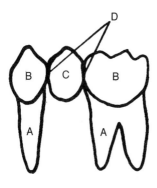

Figure 1–1

133. What type of restoration is used to reinforce an endodontically treated tooth before a crown is fabricated?
   A. An acrylic core
   B. A copper band
   C. An aluminum shell
   D. A gold post

134. Cantilever bridges
   A. are the most common bridges made
   B. are used only to replace molars
   C. always use three abutments
   D. have abutments on only one side

135. The primary function of a temporary bridge is
   A. to assist in final shade selection
   B. to help move teeth
   C. to protect teeth from thermal and contact sensitivity
   D. to improve occlusion

136. Epinephrine-impregnated cord is used to
   A. stimulate a patient who has fainted
   B. dry the prepared tooth
   C. tie stone dies together
   D. stop gingival bleeding and retract the gingiva

137. The function of the periodontium is to
   A. prevent caries
   B. support the teeth
   C. prevent vertical food impaction
   D. aid the tongue in cleansing the teeth

138. What is gingivitis?
   A. Inflammation of the soft tissues surrounding the teeth
   B. Inflammation of the cortical bone
   C. Inflammation of the teeth
   D. Inflammation around the apical foramen

139. What is periodontitis?
   A. Inflammation of the soft tissue that surrounds the teeth
   B. Inflammation of the teeth

    C. The stage of periodontal disease involving loss of bone that supports the teeth

    D. The removal of soft tooth-accumulated material

140. Another name for Vincent's disease is
    A. acute necrotizing ulcerative gingivitis
    B. acute ear infection
    C. aphthous ulcer
    D. herpetic lesions

141. A furcation in periodontics refers to
    A. a surgical procedure
    B. mobility of anterior teeth
    C. the radicular area of multirooted teeth
    D. a dry mouth

142. A splint is an appliance that
    A. holds broken teeth together
    B. connects and stabilizes mobile teeth
    C. holds soft tissue against bone
    D. keeps sutures covered after surgery

143. To correct a diastema or incisal fracture
    A. an acrylic plastic is applied
    B. orthodontic treatment is required
    C. enamel bonding materials are utilized
    D. bleaching the tooth is necessary

144. Osteoplasty is the
    A. recontouring of gingival tissue
    B. recontouring of bony defects
    C. implanting of bone
    D. treatment of choice in gingivitis

145. Gingivectomy is the
    A. surgical removal of the mucogingival junction
    B. surgical removal of the apex of a tissue
    C. replacement of inflamed gingival tissue
    D. surgical elimination of the gingival pocket

146. An abscess is
   A. a collection of serous fluid
   B. a pathway for fluid drainage
   C. a localized collection of pus
   D. always infrabony in nature

147. Drugs that are used for the relief of pain of low intensity are classified as
   A. hypnotics
   B. sedatives
   C. analgesics
   D. narcotics

148. If you had an emergency in the office involving syncope what would you be treating?
   A. Headache
   B. Hyperventilation
   C. Cardiac arrest
   D. Fainting

149. A patient having an angina attack suffers from what medical problem?
   A. Diabetes
   B. A heart condition
   C. High blood pressure
   D. Fever

150. Which of the following is most descriptive of someone in shock?
   A. Face pale, strong pulse, breathing regular
   B. Nervousness, face flushed, pulse rapid
   C. Skin cool and clammy, weak pulse, breathing irregular
   D. Nausea, rapid breathing, strong pulse

DIRECTIONS (Questions 151–180): Match the instruments in Column A with their primary function in Column B.

COLUMN A **COLUMN B**

151. broach _____
152. reamer _____
153. Luer-Lok syringe _____
154. paper-point _____
155. plugger _____

A. absorbs moisture in the root canal
B. extirpates the pulpal contents
C. carries irrigating solution to the canal
D. gains entrance and cleanses the root canal
E. assists in condensing gutta-percha into the canal

COLUMN A **COLUMN B**

156. matrix band _____
157. gingival margin trimmer _____
158. amalgam condenser _____
159. cleoid-discoid carver _____
160. amalgam carrier _____

A. compresses amalgam into the cavity preparation
B. limits the filling material to the confines of the tooth
C. places amalgam into the cavity preparation
D. carves the restoration
E. removes undermined enamel

COLUMN A **COLUMN B**

161. ultrasonic scaler _____
162. curette _____
163. sickle scaler _____
164. periodontal probe _____
165. rubber cup _____

A. hand instrument used to remove supragingival calculus
B. measures the depth of peridontal pocket
C. removes crevicular epithelium, and calculus
D. used to coronal polish all surfaces of teeth
E. vibrating instrument that knocks debris off teeth

COLUMN A   **COLUMN B**

166. heatless stone   _____   A. smooths roughness in metals
167. rag wheel   _____   B. grossly reduces an acrylic pros-
168. mandrel   _____   thesis
169. vulcanite bur   _____   C. holds unmounted stones
170. rubber wheel   _____   D. polishes acrylic prosthesis with
                                          pumice
                                      E. grossly reduces a metal prosthesis

COLUMN A   **COLUMN B**

171. plastic instrument _____   A. helps seat crowns
172. locking college   B. holds medicated cotton pledgets
     pliers   _____   C. inserts composite filling material
173. leather mallet   _____   D. carries alginate impression ma-
174. chisel   _____   terial
175. rim-lock tray   _____   E. removes unsupported enamel

COLUMN A   **COLUMN B**

176. bur No. 8   _____   A. tapered fissure bur
177. bur No. 33   _____   B. cross-cut fissure bur
178. bur No. 57   _____   C. inverted cone bur
179. bur No. 558   _____   D. small round bur
180. bur No. 1/2   _____   E. large round bur

DIRECTIONS (Questions 181–184): Match the lettered illustrations
in Figure 1–2 with the corresponding questions.

---

181. Identify the curette, periodontal probe, and syringe.
     A. B, D, and F
     B. C, J, and N
     C. I, K, and M
     D. O, H, and A

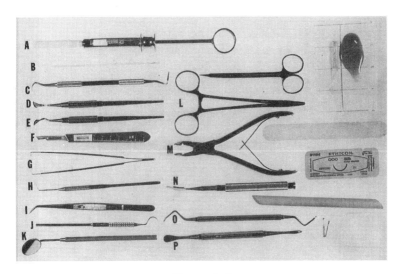

Figure 1–2

182. Identify the interproximal knife, pocket marker, and locked college pliers.
   A. C, G, and I
   B. E, J, and O
   C. G, K, and M
   D. L, M, and P

183. Identify the ronguers, scalpel, and topical anesthetic applicator.
   A. C, J, and E
   B. I, L, and D
   C. M, F, and B
   D. O, K, and N

184. Identify the needle holder, periosteal elevator, and bone chisel.
   A. C, O, and M
   B. E, J, and K
   C. G, D, and H
   D. L, P, and N

DIRECTIONS (Question 185–187): Match the lettered illustrations in Figure 1–3 with the corresponding questions.

185. Identify the plastic instrument, stainless steel crowns, and spatula.
    A. B, K, and C
    B. D, J, and G
    C. H, E, and K
    D. A, F, and B

186. Identify the base applicator, dappen dish, and locking pliers.
    A. B, K, and C
    B. D, J, and G
    C. H, E, and K
    D. A, F, and B

187. Identify the explorer, spoon excavator, and crown and collar scissors.
    A. B, D, and E
    B. D, E, and F
    C. H, F, and E
    D. A, F, and G

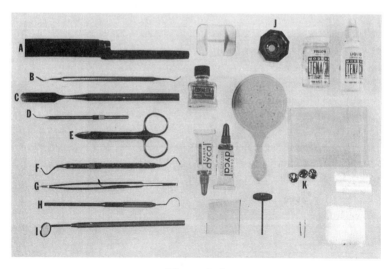

Figure 1–3

DIRECTIONS (Questions 188–190): Match the lettered illustrations in Figure 1–4 with the corresponding questions.

188. Identify the anterior rubber dam clamp, high volume evacuation tip, and rubber dam frame.
   A. G, B, and F
   B. H, E, and D
   C. J, C, and A
   D. K, D, and B

189. Identify the rubber dam punch, rubber dam clamp forceps, and premolar rubber dam clamp.
   A. A, F, and G
   B. B, C, and I
   C. C, D, and H
   D. E, A, and J

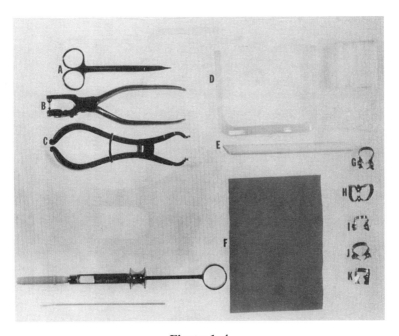

Figure 1–4

190. Identify the rubber dam, scissors, and No. 26 molar rubber dam clamp.
  A. F, A, and K
  B. G, H, and F
  C. C, D, and J
  D. D, B, and J

DIRECTIONS (Questions 191–192): Match the lettered illustrations in Figure 1–5 with the corresponding questions.

---

191. Identify the vulcanite burs, rubber impression syringe, and retraction cord.
  A. A, B, and I
  B. D, C, and E
  C. H, G, and B
  D. I, A, and C

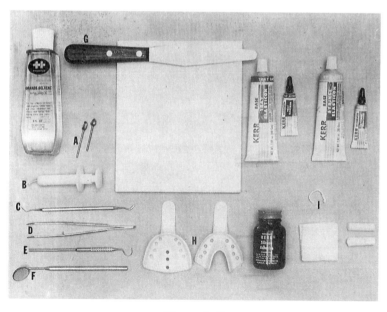

Figure 1–5

192. Identify the retraction instrument, spatula, and perforated trays.
- **A.** A, G, and H
- **B.** C, I, and G
- **C.** C, G, and H
- **D.** E, C, and I

DIRECTIONS (Questions 193–194): Match the lettered illustrations in Figure 1–6 with the corresponding questions.

---

193. Identify the composite finishing burs, composite matrices, and straight chisel.
- **A.** I, M, and J
- **B.** E, D, and H
- **C.** C, G, and F
- **D.** M, B, and H

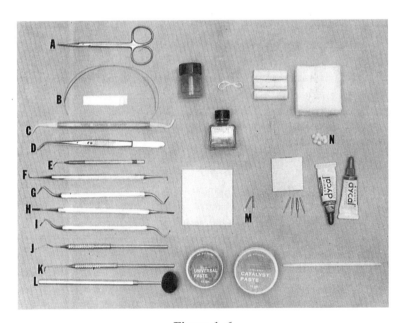

Figure 1–6

194. Identify the composite placement instrument, enamel hoe, and No. 17 explorer.
   A. C, G, and J
   B. F, D, and K
   C. H, A, and I
   D. J, B, and E

DIRECTIONS (Questions 195–206): Read each item in the charting exercise and record it on the dental chart provided (Fig. 1–7). Any type of symbol or abbreviation may be used to chart conditions. Do not use words. Refer only to the dental chart you have completed when answering the charting questions (195–206).

EXERCISE 1: Charting Items
   1. The maxillary right third molar is missing.
   2. There is a fixed bridge between the maxillary right first premolar and the maxillary right second molar.
   3. The maxillary right second premolar and first molar are missing.
   4. The maxillary right lateral incisor has a Class III mesial composite restoration present.
   5. The maxillary right central incisor has Class III distal decay.
   6. The maxillary left canine has a porcelain jacket.
   7. The maxillary left second premolar has distal occlusal decay.
   8. The maxillary left second molar has a mesial occlusal distal amalgam restoration present.
   9. There is a 6 mm periodontal pocket between the maxillary left second and third molars.
   10. The mandibular left third molar is vertically impacted.
   11. The mandibular left first molar has mesial occlusal decay and a Class III periodontal buccal furcation.
   12. The mandibular left first premolar has Class V buccal decay and Class II periodontal mobility.
   13. The mandibular left second premolar is missing and has a retained primary second molar.
   14. There is a fixed bridge between the mandibular left canine and the mandibular right canine. The mandibular left central and lateral and the mandibular right central and lateral are missing.

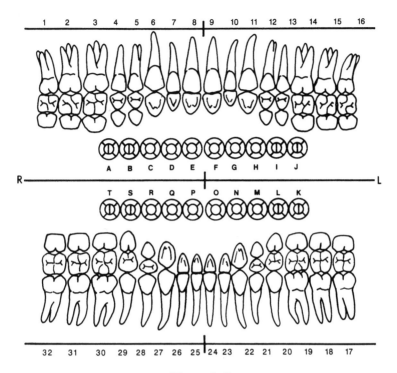

Figure 1–7

Charting Items (continued)

15. The mandibular right first premolar is not present.
16. The mandibular right second molar has a mesial occlusal distal amalgam restoration that must be replaced.

EXERCISE 1: Charting Questions

195. How many teeth are missing?
   A. 2
   B. 4
   C. 6
   D. 8

196. How many surfaces of teeth need restorations in the mandibular arch?
  A. 2
  B. 4
  C. 6
  D. 8

197. Which tooth is impacted?
  A. Mandibular left third molar
  B. Maxillary right third molar
  C. Maxillary left third molar
  D. Mandibular left second primary molar

198. What is the classification of the cavity restoration on the maxillary right lateral incisor?
  A. Class I
  B. Class II
  C. Class III
  D. Class V

199. How many surfaces of amalgam restorations are present in the maxillary and mandibular arches?
  A. 2
  B. 4
  C. 6
  D. 8

200. Where is the periodontal pocket located?
  A. Between the maxillary right second and third molars
  B. Between the maxillary left second and third molars
  C. Distal to the mandibular left first molar
  D. Between the mandibular right canine and second premolar

201. Which teeth are abutments for a fixed bridge in the mandibular arch?
  A. Mandibular right and left canines
  B. Mandibular right canine and second premolar
  C. Mandibular left canine and first premolar
  D. Mandibular lateral incisors

202. What condition exists on the maxillary left canine?
   A. Full gold crown
   B. Porcelain jacket
   C. Three-quarter crown
   D. Gold inlay

203. Which tooth has a restoration that must be replaced?
   A. Maxillary left central incisor
   B. Maxillary left second molar
   C. Mandibular right second molar
   D. Mandibular right third molar

204. What condition exists on the mandibular left first premolar?
   A. Class II caries
   B. Class V buccal caries
   C. Class V buccal composite
   D. Has a retained primary molar

205. Where is the periodontal furcation located?
   A. Maxillary right second molar buccal aspect
   B. Maxillary left second molar buccal aspect
   C. Maxillary left third molar buccal aspect
   D. Mandibular left first molar buccal aspect

206. What periodontal condition exists on the mandibular left first premolar?
   A. Class II mobility
   B. Periodontal pocket of 6 mm
   C. Periodontal furcation involvement
   D. No periodontal condition exists

Practice Test Questions 1: Chairside Assisting

Answers and Discussion

1. **(A)** A complete medical history is required before rendering any type of dental treatment on a patient. Potential life-threatening situations can be avoided by being alert to medical complications identified from a medical health questionnaire. The medical history provides information regarding premedication requirements, heart conditions, infectious diseases, allergies, and other related illnesses that are critical for the dental assistant to acknowledge before seating the patient for dental treatment.

2. **(C)** The main role of the assistant in preventive dentistry is to educate and motivate patients. The information offered usually includes material about plaque control and proper nutrition.

3. **(B)** Before applying a topical fluoride gel, the assistant must dry the teeth thoroughly. Special attention to drying occlusal surfaces is recommended, since these areas are most susceptible to dental caries.

4. **(D)** Teeth most likely to benefit from the application of pit and fissure sealants include posterior teeth with deep pits and fissures.

5. **(D)**   The assistant's eye level is 4–6″ above the dentist's eye level. This permits the assistant to have maximum visibility of the operating field and not interfere with the dentist's visibility.

6. **(A)**   When working on the lower right molars, the operator is in the 9 o'clock position, and the assistant retracts the tongue as the operator retracts the right cheek. The operator working on the lower left quadrant retracts the tongue while the assistant retracts the left cheek.

7. **(D)**   Protective barriers are necessary when sterilizing instruments. Heavy-duty utility gloves should be worn when handling soiled armamentarium and scrubbing instruments before sterilization. A face mask and safety glasses also may be used.

8. **(B)**   During the preliminary collection of clinical data the patient is observed for signs of anxiety and abnormal conditions resulting in deteriorating physical health. Poor nutrition and lesions of the oral cavity are often associated with substance abuse. The patient's insurance coverage is not part of the assessment phase process.

9. **(B)**   When working in the anterior area of the mouth, the suction tip is placed on the opposite side of the tooth being prepared and parallel to the labial or lingual surface of the tooth being prepared.

10. **(C)**   Angle's classification of malocclusion is based on the relationship between the maxillary and mandibular first molars. When the teeth are in normal occlusion (Class I neutroclusion), the mesiobuccal cusp of the maxillary molar fits in the buccal groove of the mandibular first molar. Deviations of occlusion classification include: the mandibular molars are one cusp distal to their normal position (Class II distoclusion) and the mandibular molars are one cusp mesial to their normal position (Class III mesioclusion).

11. **(A)**   A normal reading for blood pressure is 120 for systolic pressure and 80 for diastolic pressure. The reading when monitored is recorded as a fraction: 120/80. Vital signs should be monitored routinely before dental treatment and recorded in the patient's dental record.

12. (C) The purpose of aspiration is to find out if the lumen of the needle is in a blood vessel. If blood is aspirated, the needle is moved to another location before the local anesthetic is deposited.

13. (B) The condition in which a patient lacks oxygen is called hypoxia. Hypoxia is reduced oxygen within the circulatory system.

14. (B) The patient's clinical record must include an updated medical health questionnaire. The medical health questionnaire should be reviewed and updated periodically as indicated by office policy. The date and signature of the patient are also required. Potential medical emergencies can be avoided by reviewing the medical history of each patient before treatment. Legal requirements for the health professional necessitate accurate clinical record keeping, including updated medical health questionnaires on every patient. The signature of the reviewing clinician is also required on the form.

15. (A) When transferring an instrument, the assistant holds it between the thumb and forefinger, parallel to the instrument being used, close to the operating field, and opposite the working end, which is pointed toward the surface at which it will be used.

16. (D) The fulcrum digit used in the modified pen grasp is the fourth finger, or ring finger. A fulcrum serves as the pivotal point or support for stabilizing a particular finger rest.

17. (C) Class I caries is classified according to G.V. Black as cavities that occur on the occlusal surfaces of premolars and molars. Pits or fissures on the lingual surfaces of incisors near the cingulum also are classified as Class I caries.

18. (B) A denture is relined to improve the readaptation of the denture base to the underlying tissue. The procedure is made necessary by the resorption of bone in the denture-supporting area.

19. (C) The matrix band is removed slowly and carefully teased off the tooth in an occlusal direction. As the matrix band becomes free, the marginal ridge of the amalgam restoration must be held in place with an instrument to avoid accidental fracture of the restoration during matrix band removal procedures.

20. (A) The color of the nitrous oxide cylinder tank is always blue. The color blue identifies the cylinder as containing nitrous oxide gas. Nitrous oxide gas is nonflammable and is used as an inhalation agent.

21. (C) If a patient jumps out of the chair after being treated in a supine position, he or she will not have an opportunity to regain circulatory equilibrium. This can cause fainting due to lack of blood flowing to the brain.

22. (B) Irreversible hydrocolloid is loaded in a perforated tray with most of the material placed anteriorly.

23. (B) Class II cavity preparations include the occlusal and one or two proximal surfaces of premolars and molars.

24. (B) When placing a rubber dam, a blunt type of instrument may be used to invert the dam around the teeth being prepared. Inversion of the dam places the free edge of the dam into the gingival sulcus and thereby prevents leakage.

25. (C) The rubber dam napkin is used to avoid irritation around the patient's mouth by absorbing fluids and avoiding direct contact of the rubber dam with the patient's face.

26. (D) A lubricant can be placed around the holes punched in the rubber dam to facilitate the placement of the rubber dam between the teeth. A lubricant also can be used at the corners of the patient's mouth to help avoid irritation.

27. (D) Class IV cavity preparations involve the proximal surface and the incisal angle of incisors and canines.

28. (C) Debridement of the cavity preparation refers to cleaning and drying the preparation. This is accomplished by washing the preparation with water or hydrogen peroxide, followed by drying the preparation with intermittent blasts of air.

29. (A) Impression waxes are used to record bite registrations and as impression material for nonundercut areas.

30. (A) The rubber dam is removed after condensation of a Class II amalgam preparation in order to check the patient's occlusion.

31. (B) Burnishers are not used to evaluate amalgam restorations. They are used to adapt restorative materials, such as amalgam and gold foil, to the margins of the cavity preparation.

32. (C) When applying a rubber dam, the anchor tooth (tooth that is clamped) selected is 1 or 2 teeth distal to the tooth being prepared.

33. (A) Before removing the rubber dam clamp, the interseptal rubber dam material is cut carefully by stretching the rubber dam material toward the operator and cutting away from the gingiva with crown and collar scissors.

34. (D) The following pieces of equipment should be disinfected after treatment of each patient: light handles, chair controls, countertops, and chair headrest. Handpieces, curettes, and filmholders must be sterilized.

35. (B) The purpose of palpating the neck of a patient is to feel for enlarged lymph nodes, which may indicate a localized dental infection in the oral cavity or face and neck area. The lymph nodes are palpated either bidigitally or bimanually during an extraoral examination and are located on either side of the neck and under the chin. As part of the body's immune system, the lymph nodes become filled with lymphocytes to fight the foreign bodies causing the infection. The increased number of lymphocytes in one localized area results in tender, swollen nodes.

36. (A) Dental plaque is a soft white deposit that collects around the gingival margins of teeth. The bacteria in plaque are directly responsible for dental caries and gingival disease. Calculus is classified as a hard deposit, and leukoplakia refers to whitish lesions of the oral mucosa.

37. (A) Coronal polishing procedures require the use of a bristle brush attached to the dental handpiece to effectively remove soft deposits from the pits and fissured grooves of the occlusal surfaces. The rubber polishing cup may be used on all other surfaces of the teeth.

38. (D) Steam sterilization (autoclave) is the best method of sterilization because it provides the largest margin of safety by effectively destroying the hepatitis B virus. All autoclaves and chemiclaves must be biologically monitored on a periodic basis to ensure continued effective sterilization of instruments and destruction of infectious pathogens. All health care workers who are exposed frequently to blood or other body fluids should be immunized with the hepatitis B vaccine as an additional safety measure from occupational exposure to blood-borne pathogens. Appropriate disposal methods for infectious waste must also be enforced.

39. (D) To prevent a mouth mirror from fogging, gently rub the face of the mouth mirror against the buccal mucosa to coat it with a thin, transparent film of saliva.

40. (C) A cavity varnish (liner) is applied to all surfaces, including the walls and floor of a cavity preparation. The thin liquid varnish is composed of a resin base suspended in an organic solvent.

41. (D) Calcium hydroxide is used because it stimulates the formation of secondary dentin. When used as a liner in a cavity preparation, calcium hydroxide does not aid in reducing marginal leakage around the restoration because the application site is limited to the deepest portion of the cavity preparation only. The lining material does not seal dentinal tubules or provide sufficient thermal insulation.

42. (B) To prevent gagging or excess flow of alginate impression material down the back of the throat, the patient should be seated in an upright position with the head tilted slightly forward.

43. (B) The appropriate trays for obtaining alginate impressions are perforated Rim-lock (autoclavable) trays or perforated plastic (disposable) trays. Water-cooled trays are used for final hydrocolloid impressions, and styrofoam disposable trays are used for fluoride treatments. Custom-made dental compound trays are best suited for edentulous impressions with a zinc-oxide eugenol impression paste material.

44. (C) Composite resin materials must be mixed using a folding motion with a plastic type of spatula only. Metal mixing spatulas tend to discolor the resin material and are contraindicated. Placement procedures for composite resins also require the use of plastic application instruments.

45. **(A)** Criteria for a properly placed wedge (either wooden or plastic) require that the wedge ensure stability of the matrix band and separate the adjacent teeth slightly.

46. **(C)** The matrix band best suited for molars with deep gingival preparations is the metal molar band with wide gingival extensions.

47. **(A)** A Tofflemire matrix properly prepared for the mandibular right quadrant also can be used in the maxillary left quadrant. If prepared for the mandibular left quadrant, the Tofflemire matrix may be adapted also to the maxillary right quadrant.

48. **(B)** The best way to prevent gagging during impression taking is to seat the patient in an upright position with the head tilted slightly forward. Ask the patient to breathe normally through the nose. Do not overfill the tray with impression material to prevent an excess flow down into the oropharnyx area. Talk to the patient in a reassuring positive manner during the procedure to further relax the patient with a high gag reflex. It is best to take the lower impression first and the upper arch last. Cold water will retard the set and prolong the procedure. A fast set impression mix is recommended to reduce chair time for the patient.

49. **(D)** Fogged x-ray films have an overall graying image on the processed film. This is due to the use of outdated films, stray radiation, or exposure to light in the darkroom.

50. **(B)** All dental personnel working with dental x-ray equipment should wear a radiation detection badge to estimate the radiation absorbed by the wearer. The film badge is worn during x-ray exposure procedures and removed at either weekly, biweekly, or monthly intervals for evaluation.

51. **(C)** A topical anesthetic is used before administration of a local anesthetic injection for temporary surface numbness of the oral tissues. The oral tissue is dried with a 2 × 2 gauze before applying the topical anesthetic agent.

52. (B) A temporary filling is best packed (filled) with a condenser type of instrument. The appropriate condenser should be selected to adapt to the size of the cavity preparation.

53. (D) The best instruments for removing excess cement from teeth are a scaler and an explorer. Dental floss is effective for removing residual cement debris from interproximal surfaces. A knot may be formed in the dental floss before running the floss interproximally for removal of embedded deposits.

54. (C) Protective visible light eyewear is required to protect the eyes from retinal damage.

55. (A) When placing a temporary filling, it is not important to carve detailed anatomy, since the filling material is not permanent and will need to be replaced in a short period of time. Occlusion should be functional and checked before dismissing the patient. Margins must be sealed and a proper contact maintained.

56. (B) The primary use of a matrix band is to provide the missing wall in a proximal surface cavity.

57. (C) A properly placed Tofflemire matrix band should be placed at least 2 mm above the occlusal ridge to ensure proper contour and occlusion of the final restoration. The matrix band also extends 1 mm beyond the gingival margin of the preparation to ensure an appropriate seal at the base of the preparation without impinging on the actual cavity preparation, which may lead to a final restoration with inadequate or open gingival margins.

58. (C) Dental stone is used to construct models used in constructing dentures, bite plates, and bite guards.

59. (D) The beavertail burnisher is not a hand cutting instrument. The primary function of a burnishing instrument is to smooth out a metal surface while it is still malleable. The spoon excavator is used to remove soft carious dentin from a cavity preparation, and the hoe and gingival margin trimmer are used to bevel and redefine a cavity preparation.

60. (D) When assembling a Tofflemire matrix retainer, the diagonal slot should always face toward the gingival tissue.

61. (C) Wet agents cause less frictional heat than do dry agents. A suitable wet agent for flour of pumice may include water, glycerin, or mouthwash.

62. (D) Light pressure is used during coronal polishing procedures to avoid any unnecessary frictional heat, which may cause injury to the dental pulp.

63. (A) Extrinsic stains of the teeth are removed during coronal polishing procedures. Blackline stain is an extrinsic stain that often occurs around the cervical surfaces of maxillary and mandibular molars.

64. (B) Tin oxide is a white powder polishing agent for metallic restorations. Water is added to the powder to reduce frictional heat to the teeth during polishing procedures.

65. (D) Bleaching of teeth may be done in-office on teeth that have discolorations due to intrinsic staining such as tetracycline stains or mottled enamel.

66. (C) A safety precaution that may be used during application of a rubber dam clamp is to loop a strand of dental floss around the bow of the clamp, then secure the floss by tightening. This safety measure will assist in quickly retrieving the clamp should it become dislodged during the application phase of rubber dam placement.

67. (A) When seating a rubber dam clamp, the lingual jaws are placed first, then the buccal jaws are adapted. A properly placed clamp should be stable and not impinge on soft gingival tissues.

68. (D) Acidulated phosphate fluoride gel is the most common form of fluoride used with the rigid tray system. The gel is dispensed into the trays, and the patient is instructed to close and bite once the tray has been properly seated to allow the gel to penetrate and saturate all occlusal tooth surfaces. Sodium fluoride and stannous fluoride frequently are in a liquid form or rinse.

69. (B) Before applying a vitalometer to the teeth, it is necessary to dry the teeth with a 2 × 2 gauze or cotton roll. The vitalometer should contact the enamel surface only and is not recommended on metallic restorations. The vitalometer is used to determine (test) the vitality or life of a tooth. Small electrical impulses are conducted by adjusting the vitalometer monitor dial. A low reading (1–2) indicates pulpal vitality, and a high reading (9–10) indicates degeneration of the pulp, or pulpal death.

70. (A) A very low reading (1–2) on the vitalometer indicates pulpal hyperemia. Hyperemia indicates an increase in the amount of blood in the vessels of the pulp cavity. This may be due to an inflammatory process or an irritation to the pulp.

71. (C) A high reading (10) on an electric pulp tester (vitalometer) indicates that the tooth is nonvital.

72. (D) Before placing an x-ray film in the patient's mouth, it is not necessary to chart the existing restorations of the patient. A visual oral inspection of the soft tissue is recommended to aid the assistant in appropriate film size selection and film placement principles. Always place a lead apron on the patient before exposure and remove any appliances from the patient's mouth.

73. (B) Obtaining a measurement (or length) of the root canal will avoid the possibility of irritating periapical tissues by overextending instruments beyond the apex of the root. Measurement is obtained by placing a reamer in the canal and taking a radiograph.

74. (A) Three endodontic instruments are used in the root canals: files are used to enlarge and shape the canal, broaches are used to remove pulpal tissue from the canal, and reamers are used to check the path and length of the canal.

75. (C) The material commonly used to fill root canals is gutta-percha.

76. (B) A dilute sodium hypochlorite solution, such as household bleach, is recommended for cleaning dentures. The technique is known as immersion.

77. (C) Each state legislature has enacted a state Dental Practice Act, which defines the duties, responsibilities, and restrictions of the dental assistant and dentist. The state Dental Practice Act serves as a regulatory body, which monitors the practice of dentistry in the state. The Dental Board of Examiners for each individual state is appointed to interpret and enforce the regulations of the state Dental Practice Act.

78. (B) The removal of the coronal portion of the pulp is called pulpotomy. In pedodontics, there are several types of pulpal therapies possible: direct pulp capping, in which a small exposure of a vital pulp is medicated with calcium hydroxide; indirect pulp capping, in which dentin affected by the carious process is medicated with calcium hydroxide or zinc oxide-eugenol; and pulpectomy, which is complete removal of a necrotic pulp and filling of the root canals with an inert material.

79. (C) A stainless steel crown usually is indicated for full coverage of a deciduous molar. This restoration is less expensive and easier to construct than a cast gold restoration. It protects the deciduous molar, enabling it to function and permitting normal eruption of the succedaneous tooth.

80. (D) An apicoectomy is the surgical removal of the apex of the root. The procedure consists of flapping the gingival tissue over the designated area and removing bone to gain access to the root apex. The operator then cuts the root apex off and curettes the periapical infection. The flap is then sutured closed over the designated area.

81. (C) Hemisection is performed when the periodontal condition of one root threatens the survival of the tooth. Hemisection requires that root canal therapy be performed before surgical removal of a root.

82. (D) A dry socket (alveolar osteitis) is a breakdown of a blood clot in an extraction socket. It may be caused by infection, poor blood supply to the area, excessive trauma during extraction, or improper postoperative care. Treatment of a dry socket consists of irrigation of the socket and packing it with gauze and an anodyne.

83. (C) Application of direct pressure is the best technique to stop bleeding after extractions. Direct pressure is applied by having the patient bite on a gauze compress, which is placed directly over the extraction site for 30 to 45 min. This process leads to formation of a blood clot in the extraction site, which is the first step in healing.

84. (D) Rinsing with warm salt water decreases the number of microorganisms in the mouth and thereby promotes healing and helps prevent infection.

85. (A) A suture material that is resorbed by the body is gut.

86. (B) Postextraction dressings are removed and changed every 1 to 2 days as needed or until healing occurs. A postextraction dressing is used to soothe a painful condition known as alveolar osteitis, or dry socket, that may occur after the extraction of a tooth. The tooth socket is cleansed, irrigated, dried, and then packed with a medicated surgical gauze or Gelfoam. This procedure is repeated as often as necessary.

87. (C) When removing sutures, never pull the knot through the tissues. Single interrupted sutures are removed with sterile suture scissors and a pair of cotton pliers. The area is first cleansed gently with a swab dipped in peroxide to remove surface plaque and debris that have collected over the suture material. Grasp the suture with cotton pliers just below the knot and snip the suture with scissors. Gently pull through tissue. Continuous sutures require several small cuts before removal. The patient is allowed to rinse with warm water, and appropriate postoperative hygiene instructions must be given before dismissing the patient.

88. (D) In treatment of a dry socket, the alveolus may be irrigated with a warm saline solution or hydrogen peroxide and warm water.

89. (B) When placing a periodontal dressing, it is necessary to festoon the material around the neck of each tooth. The dressing material should not be excessively bulky or extend into the vestibule areas of the oral cavity. For aesthetic purposes, the dressing material should closely follow the natural contours of the dentition and not overextend onto the labial, buccal, or lingual surfaces of the teeth.

90. (C) Following periodontal surgery, the patient is instructed to omit hot, spicy, or sticky foods. All alcohol and tobacco products should be avoided, since they interfere with healing. Foods that have high nutritional value and are rich in protein are recommended to promote healing. Oral hygiene instructions include the use of a soft toothbrush dipped in water to clean off surface debris from the dressing. Disclosing agents are contraindicated during this postoperative healing time period.

91. (A) The beaks of the cotton pliers are used to gently remove a periodontal dressing. Suture removal scissors may be used to trim suture material that may become enmeshed in the periodontal dressing material.

92. (B) The assistant prepares the syringe by placing the carpule in the syringe, placing the needle on the syringe, engaging the stylet in the rubber plunger of the carpule, loosening the needle cover, and testing the syringe to be sure the anesthetic comes out. The assistant does not place the anesthetic solution in the carpule.

93. (A) Incision and drainage are used to treat a periodontal abscess. A periodontal abscess, part of the body's defense mechanism, forms when a foreign body, food, calculus, or other particle becomes lodged in a periodontal pocket.

94. (B) The terms relative analgesia or analgesia are used to identify nitrous oxide, an inhalation sedation drug. Nitrous oxide is effective in reducing anxiety during dental treatment. The inhalation agent is easy to administer and allows for rapid recovery. Indications for use of nitrous oxide sedation may include to control gagging, to raise pain threshold, to reduce fear and anxiety concerning dental treatment, to stabilize blood pressure in patients with a history of hypertension, and to control excess salivary flow.

95. (D) A patient receiving the proper level of nitrous oxide will be conscious and relaxed and have normal pupils. The administration of nitrous oxide tends to lower the blood pressure slightly.

96. (B) During the induction phase of nitrous oxide administration, the patient is given approximately 5 to 8 liters of oxygen for 1 to 2 min. The patient is instructed to breathe deeply once the nose piece is in place. Nitrous oxide is administered at the rate of 1 liter per min. while the oxygen flow is decreased by 1 liter intervals in the same manner. Vital signs must be monitored before the induction phase.

97. (A) Instructing the patient to hold his or her breath for 30 seconds, then inhale deeply is not the correct procedure for the induction phase of nitrous oxide sedation.

98. (C) If the patient exhibits signs and symptoms of the excitement stage of nitrous oxide sedation, the nitrous flow must be decreased immediately. The objective of nitrous oxide sedation is to achieve a baseline level of sedation such that dental treatment may be administered in a relaxed setting with as little discomfort to the patient as possible. Preexcitement or excitement signs and symptoms exhibited by the patient may include giddiness, laughter, tingling sensations in hands and feet, and difficulty in communication.

99. (C) The flowmeter controls the volume of gas administered to the patient. The flow of each gas—oxygen and nitrous oxygen—is indicated in liters per minute when regulated by the control dials. By observing the positions of the floats in the flowmeter columns of each cylinder gauge, it is possible for the operator to determine the appropriate volume of gas necessary for effective sedation and dental treatment.

100. (D) The dental assistant may not administer nitrous oxide to a patient if requested to do so by the patient. Under the doctor's direct supervision and orders, the dental assistant may assist in the administration of nitrous oxide sedation. The doctor must be present at the patient's chairside during the procedure of nitrous oxide administration. The state Dental Practice Act should be consulted for further definition of the individual responsibilities and acceptable duties of the doctor and dental assistant regarding the administration of nitrous oxide.

101. (E) Study models are used as references to show progress in orthodontic cases, to help in treatment planning in all phases of dentistry, to show arch shape and arch relationship, and to help fabricate restorations, such as temporary bridges and mouth guards.

The study models show occlusal relationships and help construct custom trays. Study models may be entered as evidence in a court of law in conjunction with a malpractice suit.

102. (D) The rubber cup prophylaxis is indicated before placement of the rubber dam to avoid displacement of debris under the gingiva. By removing the plaque and other soft deposits from the teeth, application of the rubber dam is completed in a plaque-free environment. The dental floss used to seat the interseptal rubber dam material does not, therefore, force any soft debris into the gingival sulcus.

103. (A) Plaque control programs should contain oral physiotherapy instructions, nutritional counseling to decrease the intake of sugars and carbohydrates, and behavior modification techniques to motivate patients into practicing good daily oral hygiene habits. A clinical examination is performed by the doctor before implementing a plaque control program and is not a part of the patient's plaque control appointment.

104. (E) When trimming study models with a model trimmer, it is necessary to wear protective eyewear to prevent injury to the eyes. A sufficient water flow must be circulating through the model trimmer unit before use to facilitate the trimming of the plaster/stone models. When actual trimming begins, do not allow fingers to come in close contact with the trimming lathe. Begin by occluding models and start with the mandibular cast. After trimming procedures allow the cast to dry for 24 hr. before final polishing and labeling.

105. (A) The dental assistant may examine the oral cavity with a mouth mirror to chart existing restorations, missing teeth, and obvious lesions. Periodontal pockets must be measured first with a periodontal probe before charting. This procedure is performed by a doctor or a dental hygienist only.

106. (A) Functions of a good recall system may include a prophy and fluoride treatment, evaluation and examination by the dentist, and positive reinforcement of good oral hygiene habits and correction of any bad dental habits. The assistant cannot diagnose x-rays.

107. **(E)** The mouth mirror may be used to retract the buccal mucosa and tongue and to reflect or illuminate light in the oral cavity. The mouth mirror is used for indirect vision while working on the lingual surfaces of the maxillary anterior teeth and in other areas where direct vision is not possible.

108. **(D)** Protective barriers include gloves, masks, and protective eyewear. The barriers assist in controlling cross-contamination and preventing contraction of hepatitis. Subacute bacterial endocarditis is a microbial infection of the heart valves that occurs in patients with a history of valvular defects or a weakened endocardium due to congenital heart defects. The early onset of rheumatic fever often leads to permanent heart valvular damage, which may in turn lead to subacute bacterial endocarditis (SBE) if prophylactic antibiotic coverage is not administered before dental treatment. Wearing protective barriers does not prevent the contraction of SBE, angina, or epilepsy, since these illnesses are not contracted in this manner.

109. **(B)** When cementing temporary crowns, the consistency and amount of cement placed in the temporary crown depend on the type of crown to be seated. After cementation, the occlusion is checked and adjusted.

110. **(C)** During the application of pit and fissure sealants, which are polymerized by an ultraviolet light, it is necessary to use protective shaded eyewear. In order to keep the teeth as dry as possible before sealant application, a rubber dam may be applied.

111. **(A)** Glass ionomer cements are used for permanent restorations, luting procedures, and insulating bases. The powder is made from aluminosilicate glass, and the liquid is polyacrylic acid and water based. The cement exhibits physical properties of high compressive strength and adhesion to reduce marginal leakage. Secondary decay is also controlled by the ionomer cements, which incorporate fluoride in the powder composition, which is slowly leached into the enamel surface after placement.

112. **(D)** When teaching toothbrushing, the important emphasis should be on the complete and thorough removal of dental plaque regardless of brushing time.

113. (A) Hand cutting instruments used in restorative dentistry are the spoon excavator to remove carious lesions, the hoe, the hatchet, and the chisel to refine the cavity preparation, the knife and file to remove excess restorative material, and the cleoid-discoid to carve restorative material.

114. (A) A mixed dentition exists when there are deciduous and permanent teeth existing simultaneously in a child's mouth. This condition begins when the first permanent molars erupt, at age 6, and lasts until the second primary molars are exfoliated, at about age 12.

115. (C) After a topical fluoride application, the patient is instructed not to eat, rinse, or brush teeth for approximately 30 min. This allows for further penetration of the fluoride ion into the enamel.

116. (B) If a second primary molar is lost prematurely, a space maintainer is placed in the mouth to maintain the room necessary for the normal eruption of the permanent second premolar. The use of either a removable or a fixed space maintainer is dictated by the situation.

117. (C) A steady stream of warm air may desiccate the dentin and be injurious to the pulp. The correct way to dry a cavity preparation is to use cotton pledgets or short blasts of air or both.

118. (A) A back-ordered item is a supply item that currently is unavailable and will be shipped when it is available.

119. (C) Radiation exposure time for an edentulous patient should be reduced by 25%.

120. (D) The clasp of the partial denture contacts the abutment teeth. It functions to stabilize and retain the denture.

121. (A) The saddle of the partial denture contacts the edentulous ridge. Replacement teeth are placed on the saddle area.

122. (C) The function of the preliminary impression is to obtain a model on which a custom-made tray is fabricated. The custom-made tray is used to make a second and more accurate impression of the denture-bearing surface.

123. **(C)** A facebow is used to mount the upper cast on an articulator. This mounting should transfer the relationship of the maxilla to the temporomandibular joint accurately to the articulator.

124. **(A)** Wax bite blocks are used to record vertical dimension, centric relation, and facial contour and to set up denture teeth.

125. **(B)** The portion of the denture that should not be polished is the part contacting the denture-bearing mucosa. If adjustments are made on the tissue side of the denture, they can be smoothed with a small rubber wheel.

126. **(A)** To replace an intact tooth in a denture, the area on the denture where the tooth has popped out is roughened, denture repair acrylic is placed on the area, the tooth is reset, and the acrylic is allowed to set.

127. **(D)** Rubber based materials are used to make detailed final impressions. The light-body syringe material has low viscosity and the heavy-body tray material has high viscosity.

128. **(D)** An immediate denture is inserted into the patient's mouth during the same appointment in which the remaining teeth, usually anterior, are extracted. Some advantages are improved healing at the extraction sites, greater patient comfort, shorter adaptation period, improved function, and improved appearance.

129. **(C)** Tissue conditioning is used to return unhealthy tissue, caused by an ill-fitting denture, to a healthy condition. This procedure must be accomplished before final impressions are made to construct a new denture. The treatment entails placing a soft material in the patient's present denture that will permit the unhealthy tissue to recover.

130. **(A)** Shade selection is accomplished in natural light with the aid of a shade guide. The shade of the acrylic or porcelain will depend on several factors, some of which are the shade of adjacent teeth, the shade of the patient's face, and the individual teeth involved (central incisors might be lighter than canines).

131. **(B)** Fixed bridges function to prevent movement of the remaining teeth, restore function of the missing teeth, and create an aesthetic appearance.

132. **(A)** Teeth that support a fixed bridge are called abutments (Fig. 1-1A). Other parts of a fixed bridge are retainers (Fig. 1–1B), which are restorations, crowns, or inlays that are permanently cemented on abutments. Pontics (Fig. 1–1C), which are the replacements for the missing teeth and are connected to the retainers, and connectors (Fig. 1–1D), which attach the pontics and retainers.

133. **(D)** A gold post is used to reinforce an endodontically treated tooth before a crown preparation is made. Endodontically treated teeth are more brittle than are nonendodontically treated teeth. To prevent further fractures of these teeth, they should be reinforced before a crown is fabricated for them.

134. **(D)** Cantilever bridges are fixed bridges with abutments on only one side. These bridges are used for esthetics and to eliminate the need for a removable bridge.

135. **(C)** Temporary bridges are used for esthetics, mastication, decreased thermal sensitivity, stabilizing teeth, as a model for the permanent bridge, and for decreased contact sensitivity.

136. **(D)** Epinephrine-impregnated cord is used to stop gingival bleeding and to retract the gingiva before taking an impression with an elastic impression material. Epinephrine is a vasoconstrictor that stops the bleeding, and the physical presence of the cord causes the gingival retraction.

137. **(B)** The function of the periodontium is to support the teeth. Periodontal disease is the destruction of this supporting mechanism, which can lead to the loss of a tooth.

138. **(A)** Gingivitis is inflammation of the gingival tissues surrounding the teeth. The etiology is usually poor oral hygiene, which allows plaque to remain on the teeth. If treated in its early stages by removal of the irritants, the disease process is reversible.

139. **(C)** Periodontitis is a stage in periodontal disease wherein there is a destruction of bone supporting the teeth. This condition is often the extension of untreated gingival inflammation (gingivitis). If periodontitis is not treated, it will progress until teeth are lost due to lack of supporting bone. The formation of periodontal pockets also occurs with periodontal disease. A pocket is a pathologic condition that cannot be cleansed by the patient. If not eliminated, pockets usually progress and cause further destruction of the supporting apparatus of the teeth.

140. **(A)** Another name for Vincent's disease is acute necrotizing ulcerative gingivitis (or trench mouth). It is caused by poor oral hygiene, physical stress, mental stress, and smoking. The gingival tissue is red and puffy. It bleeds easily, lacks interdental papillae, is painful, and has a fetid odor.

141. **(C)** A furcation refers to the radicular area of multirooted teeth. Furcations in teeth with two roots are called bifurcations. Furcations in teeth with three roots are called trifurcations.

142. **(B)** A splint is an appliance that connects and stabilizes mobile teeth. Splints are made of various materials, including cast gold, wire, and amalgam.

143. **(C)** To correct a diastema or incisal fracture enamel bonding materials are utilized. Resin bonded bridges, veneers, and other restorative materials improve retention through bonding procedures.

144. **(B)** Osteoplasty is the recontouring of bony defects. The procedure is performed to obtain an anatomic condition that can be maintained in health by the patient.

145. **(D)** Gingivectomy is the surgical elimination of a gingival pocket so the patient can completely eliminate the plaque surrounding his or her teeth.

146. **(C)** An abscess is a localized collection of pus. The specific name of the abscess is derived from its location. It can be periapical, periodontal, pericoronal, or subperiosteal.

147. (C) Analgesics are drugs that may be used for the relief of pain of low intensity. Analgesic drugs as a rule are also antipyretics.

148. (D) Fainting is also known as syncope. Syncope is a temporary loss of consciousness due to an insufficient supply of blood to the brain. Treatment of syncope includes placing the patient in a position such that the feet are elevated higher than the head to cause the flow of blood toward the head instead of the stomach. Spirits of ammonia may be used by passing the vial just under the patient's nostrils. The ammonia vapors are strong and allow for the quick inhalation of additional oxygen. Vital signs, including pulse and blood pressure, must be monitored.

149. (B) An angina attack signals a heart problem. Angina pectoris is a painful condition of the heart caused by a lack of blood to the heart muscles. Patients with a history of angina may take special medications, such as nitroglycerin, which is administered sublingually.

150. (C) Symptoms of shock include cold, clammy skin, weak pulse, and irregular breathing. Low blood pressure is also a sign of shock.

151. (B)

152. (D)

153. (C)

154. (A)

155. (E)

156. (B)

157. (E)

158. (A)

159. (D)

160. (C)

161. (E)

162. (C)

163. (A)

164. (B)

165. (D)

166. (E)

167. (D)

168. (C)

169. (B)

170. (A)

171. (C)

172. (B)

173. (A)

174. (E)

175. (D)

176. (E)

177. (C)

178. (A)

179. (B)

180. (D)

181. (D)

182. (A)

183. (C)

184. (D)

185. (A)

186. (B)

187. (C)

188. (B)

189. (B)

190. (A)

191. (A)

192. (C)

193. (D)

194. (A)

195. (D)

196. (C)

197. (A)

198. (C)

199. (C)

200. (B)

201. (A)

202. (B)

203. (C)

204. (B)

205. (D)

206. (A)

Practice Test Questions 2: Dental Radiology

DIRECTIONS (Questions 1–100): Each of the questions or incomplete statements in this section is followed by four suggested answers or completions. Select the **ONE** lettered answer or completion that is **BEST** in each case.

---

1. A dental assistant may expose radiographs if
   A. the dentist gives permission
   B. he or she is a certified dental assistant
   C. it is permissible in the state in which he or she is employed
   D. he or she is supervised by the dentist or hygienist

2. The most sensitive cells to ionizing radiation are
   A. bone cells
   B. muscle cells
   C. nerve cells
   D. reproductive cells

3. The best type of x-ray to penetrate body tissue is
   A. low frequencies
   B. hard rays, short wavelength
   C. long wavelength
   D. soft rays, long wavelength

4. Before seating the dental patient it is necessary to cover which of the following items with disposable plastic wrap?
   A. X-ray exposure control panel
   B. Lead apron
   C. X-ray film holding devices
   D. Operator film badge

5. An exposed x-ray film covered with a plastic barrier envelope is considered to be
   A. sterile
   B. disinfected
   C. contaminated
   D. noninfectious

6. Milliamperage controls
   A. the speed with which electrons move from cathode to anode
   B. cooling of the anode
   C. heating of the anode
   D. heating of the cathode

7. The dental assistant must utilize which of the following personal protective equipment (PPE) when exposing films?
   A. Safety goggles
   B. Gloves
   C. Chin-length face shield
   D. Tinted lenses

8. The lead diaphragm determines the size and shape of the
   A. electron cloud
   B. film used
   C. x-ray beam
   D. filament

9. The portion of the target that is struck by electrons is called the
   A. focal spot
   B. photon point
   C. principal point
   D. end point

10. Proper collimation for the film size and target–film distance will
    A. increase the wavelength
    B. decrease the wavelength
    C. increase the kVp
    D. decrease the radiation received by the patient

11. To increase the penetrating quality of an x-ray beam, the auxiliary must
    A. increase kVp
    B. decrease kVp
    C. increase mA
    D. increase FFD

12. The x-ray at the center of the primary beam is called the
    A. photon ray
    B. central ray
    C. secondary ray
    D. restricted beam

13. A test for quality control relative to manual processing may be accomplished utilizing a
    A. test tube
    B. darkroom safelight
    C. water thermometer
    D. stepwedge

14. Filtration of the x-ray beam protects the patient by
    A. eliminating all radiation from the x-ray head
    B. eliminating weak wavelength x-rays from the x-ray beam
    C. eliminating short wavelength x-rays from the x-ray beam
    D. decreasing exposure time

15. Information and instructions for proper disposal of x-ray processing solutions may be found in the
    A. darkroom
    B. dental laboratory
    C. product material safety data sheet
    D. office exposure control plan

16. Scatter radiation is a type of
   A. secondary radiation
   B. primary radiation
   C. stray radiation
   D. filtered radiation

17. The quality, or penetrating power, of secondary radiation is
   A. more than that of primary radiation
   B. less than that of primary radiation
   C. the same as that of primary radiation
   D. unrelated to that of primary radiation

18. X-ray processing tanks are considered secondary containers and according to OSHA (Occupational Safety Health Administration) standards must be
   A. sealed
   B. labeled
   C. sterilized
   D. registered

19. The time period between the effects of cumulative radiation and visible tissue damage is the
   A. short-term period
   B. acute effect period
   C. latent period
   D. long-term period

20. The amount of radiation a person receives
   A. begins anew each day
   B. is cumulative only on the skin
   C. is cumulative in the entire body
   D. is not harmful in small doses

21. Maximum protection of the patient requires that the x-ray beam pass through a
   A. shielded open-ended cone
   B. plastic closed-ended cone
   C. shielded closed-ended cone
   D. lead apron

22. A technique used to measure the operator's exposure to radiation is
   A. to check the color of the operator's fingernails
   B. for the operator to wear a radiation film badge
   C. to multiply the number of films the operator has exposed by 0.1 rem
   D. to count the number of full mouth x-ray series taken

23. Accumulated radiation dosage for those who work with radiation may not exceed
   A. 0–1 rem/week
   B. 1 rem/week
   C. 10 rems/week
   D. 100 rems/week

24. To avoid exposure to secondary radiation, the operator should stand
   A. at least 6′ from the x-ray head
   B. 2′ to the right of the primary beam
   C. any distance in back of the x-ray head
   D. 4′ in front of the patient

25. The most effective way to reduce gonadal exposure from x-rays is to
   A. increase the kVp
   B. use a lead lap apron
   C. increase vertical angulation
   D. use ultraspeed film

26. After each use, the lead lap apron must be
   A. stored in the darkroom
   B. folded neatly and stored in the operatory
   C. draped over a support rod unfolded
   D. discarded for appropriate infection control

27. The best technique for reducing the radiation exposure to both patient and operator is the use of
   A. an automatic timer
   B. fast film
   C. thinner films
   D. a thicker cellulose acetate base

28. Film speed is determined by the
   A. amount of silver bromide salt
   B. thickness of cellulose acetate base
   C. size of the silver bromide crystals
   D. side of the film exposed

29. The radiographic film is covered with an emulsion of
   A. silver bromide salts
   B. cellulose
   C. silver acetate
   D. potassium bromide

30. The raised button on the radiograph aids in
   A. determining film speed
   B. processing
   C. drying
   D. mounting

31. The purpose of the lead foil in dental film is to
   A. provide stiffness to the film
   B. reduce film fogging
   C. absorb the primary beam
   D. prevent scattered radiation to the patient

32. The detection of interproximal caries is seen best with a (an)
   A. occlusal film
   B. panorex film
   C. bite-wing film
   D. lateral head plate

33. Which extraoral film is used to visualize the sinus?
   A. Water's film
   B. Lateral skull film
   C. Occlusal film
   D. Posterior–anterior film

34. X-ray films should be kept by the dentist along with other records for
   A. 1 yr.
   B. 2 yr.
   C. 5 yr.
   D. indefinitely

35. The best place to store unexposed x-ray film is in a
   A. lead container
   B. puncture resistant sealed container
   C. darkroom
   D. warm area protected from stray radiation

36. The periapical film reveals
   A. the entire jaw
   B. upper and lower teeth in the same film
   C. interproximal caries
   D. the entire tooth, including the apex

37. The principle used in panoramic radiography is
   A. long cone paralleling
   B. laminagraphy
   C. horizontal curvature
   D. panoramography

38. A material or substance that does **NOT** stop or absorb x-rays is known as
   A. radiographic
   B. radiopaque
   C. radiolucent
   D. radiodontic

39. A material or substance that **DOES** stop or absorb x-rays is known as
   A. radiographic
   B. radiopaque
   C. radiolucent
   D. radiodontic

40. All of the tissues listed are radiopaque **EXCEPT** the
   A. enamel
   B. cortical plate
   C. pulp chamber
   D. alveolar bone

41. Which of these appears radiolucent?
   A. Caries
   B. Calculus
   C. Torus
   D. Root tips

42. What is the name of the diagonal radiopaque line visible at the lower part of the roots of the mandibular molars?
 A. Mandibular canal
 B. External oblique ridge
 C. Inferior border of mandible
 D. Internal oblique line

43. What is the small circular radiolucency near the roots of the mandibular premolars called?
 A. Lingual foramen
 B. Mental foramen
 C. Mandibular foramen
 D. Incisive foramen

44. What term describes the u-shaped radiopaque structure often seen in maxillary molar films?
 A. Hamulus
 B. Tuberosity
 C. Zygoma
 D. Coronoid process

45. What is the thin radiopaque band between the maxillary incisors called?
 A. Median palatine suture
 B. Nasal septum
 C. Inverted Y
 D. Zygoma

46. What term describes the heavily radiopaque midpoint of the mandible?
 A. Zygoma
 B. Odontoma
 C. Hamulus
 D. Symphysis

47. What is the small circular radiolucency below the mandibular incisor roots called?
 A. Incisive foramen
 B. Lingual foramen
 C. Mental foramen
 D. Buccal foramen

48. What is the large radiolucent area shown on maxillary molar radiographs called?
   A. Maxillary sinus
   B. Maxillary septum
   C. Maxillary tuberosity
   D. Maxillary sequestrum

49. What is the long, narrow, and radiolucent area visible below the roots of the mandibular molars called?
   A. Inferior border
   B. Internal oblique line
   C. External oblique line
   D. Mandibular canal

50. What is the radiopaque circular area below the apices of the mandibular incisors called?
   A. Genial tubercles
   B. Mental ridge
   C. Symphysis
   D. Lamina dura

51. What is the basic principle of the bisecting the angle technique?
   A. The central ray must be directed at right angles to the tooth
   B. The central ray must be directed at right angles to the film
   C. The central ray must be directed at right angles to an imaginary line that bisects the angle formed by the long axis of the tooth and the plane of the film
   D. The central ray must be directed at a 45° angle to the embrasures

52. All of the following are basic principles of the paralleling technique **EXCEPT**
   A. the film must be parallel to the long axis of tooth
   B. an 8″ short cone must be used
   C. the source of the x-ray must be directed perpendicularly to tooth and film
   D. a 16″ extension or long cone must be used

53. When taking a full mouth series of intraoral x-rays, the sagittal plane of the patient's head should be
    A. perpendicular to the floor
    B. parallel to the floor
    C. parallel to the tube
    D. perpendicular to the central ray

54. The ala-tragus line is parallel to the floor when taking
    A. mandibular occlusal films
    B. mandibular periapical films
    C. extraoral films only
    D. maxillary periapical films

55. The occlusal plane of the maxillary arch being radiographed should be
    A. perpendicular to the floor
    B. parallel to the floor
    C. at an angle of 45° to the floor
    D. at an angle of 30° to the floor

56. Vertical angulation in the bisecting technique for the same radiograph can differ in patients because of
    A. the size of the teeth
    B. anatomic differences
    C. gagging
    D. age

57. Periapical films should extend beyond the occlusal plane
    A. 1/8″
    B. 1/4″
    C. 3/8″
    D. 1/2″

58. Firm placement of the film will help prevent
    A. overlapping
    B. foreshortening
    C. gagging
    D. elongation

59. A latent image is
   A. an image taken with a long exposure
   B. found only on fast films
   C. composed of energized silver halide crystals
   D. a very light image on the developed film

60. Cone cutting results from the central ray
   A. not being aimed at the center of film
   B. having incorrect horizontal angulation
   C. having insufficient vertical angulation
   D. being eliminated from a closed plastic cone

61. Black lines across the film may be the result of
   A. double exposure
   B. cone cutting
   C. underexposure
   D. excessive bending

62. Blurred films can result from
   A. old film
   B. movement of the patient
   C. increased kVp
   D. a faulty x-ray unit

63. If a patient is reluctant to be radiographed, the assistant should
   A. refer the patient to the dental hygienist
   B. reschedule the patient
   C. refer the patient to an x-ray laboratory
   D. explain the procedure thoroughly to the patient

64. Exposure of a radiograph on a child
   A. requires less time than on an adult
   B. requires more time than on an adult
   C. requires the same time as on an adult
   D. should never be attempted

65. Intensifying screens
   A. are used in intraoral films
   B. decrease exposure time of extraoral films
   C. create additional x-rays
   D. fuse with the film

66. As the target-film distance is increased, there is
 A. more chance of overlapping
 B. more chance of elongation
 C. less distortion
 D. more chance of foreshortening

67. A panorex film that exhibits distortion in the molar region and is lighter on one side of the film only indicates that
 A. the patient's head was not tipped down at a 5° angle
 B. the wrong caliper adjustment scale was read
 C. the patient's chin was not positioned properly
 D. a cotton roll was not placed between the anterior incisors

68. The usual number of films in a complete dentulous radiographic survey is
 A. 10–12
 B. 18–20
 C. 24–26
 D. 26–28

69. In the paralleling technique, a device used to hold the film in the patient's mouth is
 A. a film holder
 B. a plastic dental instrument
 C. the patient's finger
 D. a rubber bite block

70. Extraoral films are
 A. not sensitive to light
 B. less sensitive to light than intraoral films
 C. just as sensitive to light as intraoral films
 D. more sensitive to light than intraoral films

71. If the mA is increased while the kVp and the exposure time are kept constant, the resulting films will
 A. be lighter
 B. be darker
 C. remain the same
 D. have a herringbone pattern

72. Elongation is caused by
   A. insufficient vertical angulation
   B. too much vertical angulation
   C. insufficient horizontal angulation
   D. excessive bending of the film

73. Foreshortening is caused by
   A. insufficient vertical angulation
   B. too much vertical angulation
   C. insufficient horizontal angulation
   D. excessive bending of the film

74. If a film is exposed on the wrong side, the result will be
   A. darker films
   B. no image at all
   C. no effect
   D. a herringbone pattern

75. After a film is exposed, the target–film distance is doubled. The exposure time necessary to obtain a second film of equal density to the first film is
   A. the same as the first film
   B. twofold
   C. threefold
   D. fourfold

76. Which of the following is used to describe the blackness of an exposed radiograph?
   A. Density
   B. Detail
   C. Darkness
   D. Development

77. The difference in density of various regions of a radiograph is called
   A. collimation
   B. contrast
   C. filtration
   D. definition

78. For maximum penetration of x-rays, which of the following combinations would you select?
   A. 90 kVp and 10 mA
   B. 65 kVp and 10 mA
   C. 70 kVp and 90 mA
   D. 10 kVp and 65 mA

79. Appropriate infection control procedures during x-ray exposure should include
   A. wiping the film holders with alcohol gauze
   B. use of a thyroid collar
   C. placement of a lead screen around the patient
   D. placement of a disposable plastic wrap over the x-ray tubehead

80. Radiographs of edentulous portions of a patient's mouth
   A. should be exposed routinely
   B. should be exposed only on request of the patient
   C. should be exposed only if the entire arch is edentulous
   D. are unnecessary

81. Films left overnight in the fixer
   A. will be clear
   B. will be too dark to read
   C. will not be affected
   D. will disintegrate

82. During processing, when can radiographs safely be exposed to light?
   A. After the final wash
   B. After development
   C. After the first wash
   D. After being placed in the fixer

83. Film fog can occur if there is
   A. extremely thick bone
   B. a light leak in the darkroom
   C. slow film
   D. reversal of the film

84. Film is washed after removing it from the developing solution to
    A. remove any debris on the film
    B. speed up the developing process
    C. stop the developing process
    D. remove the precipitated silver salts

85. The fixing solution is
    A. acidic
    B. neutral
    C. basic
    D. first basic, then neutral after dilution

86. Two films are developed for the same length of time but at different temperatures. The film developed at the higher temperature will be
    A. lighter
    B. darker
    C. the same
    D. clear

87. If an unexposed film is processed, it will appear
    A. white
    B. black
    C. blue
    D. clear

88. Fixing the film
    A. removes the unaffected silver salts
    B. removes the affected silver salts
    C. softens the film
    D. peels the emulsion from the film base

89. The temperature of the radiographic processing solutions is adjusted by
    A. individual heaters
    B. chemical interaction
    C. a temperature-adjustable waterbath
    D. gas heaters

90. If a properly processed film is left overnight in the water, it will be
   A. dark
   B. light with faded image
   C. unchanged
   D. clear with no image

91. After the films are removed from the fixer, they are washed for
   A. 5–10 min.
   B. 11–19 min.
   C. 20–30 min.
   D. 1 hr.

92. For the developing chemicals to work, the solution must be
   A. acidic
   B. neutral
   C. basic
   D. very warm

93. A processed film reveals small white spots, indicating incomplete development. The error on the film during processing was caused by
   A. exposure to visible light and incomplete fixing
   B. films coming in contact with fixing solution before the proper processing procedure
   C. incomplete fixing and films not agitated in developer
   D. exposure to visible light and trapped air bubbles on film

94. Reticulation is
   A. cracking of the film emulsion
   B. an electric charge in the developing solution
   C. a latent image
   D. caused by excess radiation

95. The best way to dry processed film manually is to
   A. place films on a flat countertop with towels
   B. use the air syringe from the dental unit
   C. hang the films over the heat sterilizer
   D. hang film racks in the darkroom carefully so as not to allow wet films to contact each other

96. Films not fixed for a long enough period of time will appear
    A. to have black lines running through them
    B. to be brittle
    C. to have a brown tint
    D. white

97. The chemicals used in processing solutions are dissolved in
    A. cellulose acetate
    B. distilled water
    C. a thick emulsion
    D. potassium bromide

98. The strength of the safelight permitted in the darkroom depends on the
    A. size of the film
    B. secured lighting in the room
    C. sensitivity of the film
    D. tooth being radiographed

99. How often should the processing solutions be changed?
    A. Each week
    B. Every 3–4 weeks
    C. Every 5–6 weeks
    D. Every 7–8 weeks

100. The optimum time–temperature relationship for processing dental radiographs is
    A. $74°$ F for $4\frac{1}{2}$ min.
    B. $68°$ F for $4\frac{1}{2}$ min.
    C. $50°$ F for 5 min.
    D. $70°$ F for 6 min.

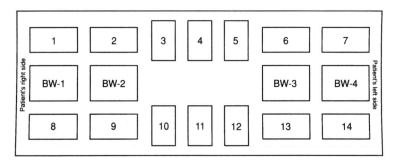

Figure 2–1

DIRECTIONS (Questions 101–118): Figure 2–1 is a mount for radiographs, with each space assigned a number. Questions 101 through 118 have assorted films to be mounted. Based on anatomic landmarks, select the correct film placement for the mount. The bubble or raised dot on each film is toward you.

101.

    A. 9
    B. 14
    C. BW-3
    D. 7
    E. BW-4

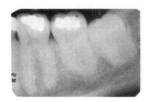

Figure 2–2

102.

    A. 3
    B. 4
    C. 11
    D. 13
    E. 10

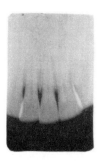

Figure 2–3

103.
   A. BW-1
   B. 8
   C. 1
   D. 6
   E. 2

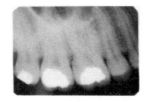

Figure 2–4

104.
   A. 12
   B. 11
   C. 5
   D. 10
   E. 9

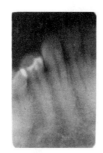

Figure 2–5

105.
   A. 1
   B. 2
   C. 6
   D. 7
   E. 13

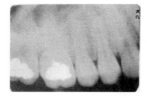

Figure 2–6

106.
   A. BW-1
   B. BW-2
   C. BW-3
   D. BW-4
   E. 8

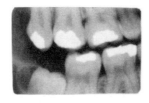

Figure 2–7

107.

    A. 3
    B. 4
    C. 5
    D. 12
    E. 11

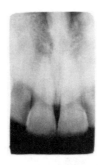

Figure 2–8

108.

    A. 1
    B. 2
    C. 6
    D. 7
    E. BW-4

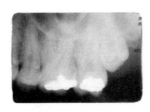

Figure 2–9

109.

    A. 3
    B. 4
    C. 5
    D. 11
    E. 10

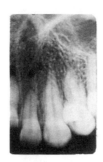

Figure 2–10

110.

    A. BW-1
    B. BW-2
    C. BW-3
    D. BW-4
    E. 1

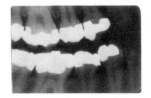

Figure 2–11

111.

- **A.** 3
- **B.** 4
- **C.** 5
- **D.** 12
- **E.** 10

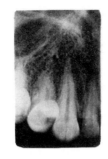

Figure 2–12

112.

- **A.** BW-1
- **B.** BW-2
- **C.** BW-3
- **D.** BW-4
- **E.** 7

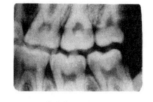

Figure 2–13

113.

- **A.** 3
- **B.** 5
- **C.** 10
- **D.** 11
- **E.** 12

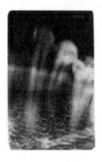

Figure 2–14

114.

- **A.** 9
- **B.** 2
- **C.** 6
- **D.** 7
- **E.** 14

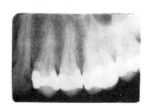

Figure 2–15

115.

    A. 9
    B. 2
    C. 13
    D. 14
    E. BW-3

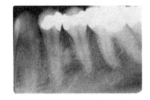

Figure 2–16

116.

    A. 8
    B. 9
    C. 6
    D. 14
    E. 13

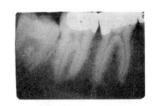

Figure 2–17

117.

    A. BW-3
    B. 2
    C. 9
    D. 7
    E. 8

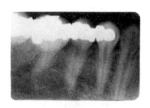

Figure 2–18

118.

    A. 1
    B. 6
    C. BW-3
    D. 8
    E. BW-1

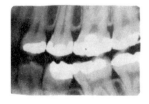

Figure 2–19

DIRECTIONS (Questions 119–141): For each of the items in this section, **ONE** or **MORE** of the numbered options is correct. Choose answer
   A. if only 1, 2, and 3 are correct
   B. if only 1 and 3 are correct
   C. if only 2 and 4 are correct
   D. if only 4 is correct
   E. if all are correct

---

119. Extraoral films are used
   1. to help diagnose fractures
   2. when a patient cannot open his or her mouth
   3. to help visualize pathologic conditions of the sinus
   4. to evaluate the position of impacted teeth

120. A maxillary molar film reveals a triangular radiopaque landmark on the lower corner of the film. The landmark visible in this film is the
   1. maxillary tuberosity
   2. maxillary sinus
   3. hamular process
   4. coronoid process of mandible

121. The dental assistant's goal in radiation protection is zero occupational exposure. This is accomplished by
   1. never holding the film for the patient
   2. always being 6′ away from the machine
   3. working in a shielded area
   4. wearing a film badge

122. In order to protect the patient from unnecessary x-ray exposure, the dental assistant should
   1. drape the patient with a lead-lined apron
   2. use good chairside techniques that will avoid retakes
   3. use high-speed film
   4. use a closed-end pointed cone x-ray tube

123. Dark films will result from
   1. underdeveloping
   2. overdeveloping
   3. underexposing
   4. overexposing

124. Light films will result from
   1. underdeveloping
   2. overdeveloping
   3. underexposure
   4. overexposure

125. Overlapping is a result of
   1. incorrect processing
   2. patient movement
   3. excessive bending of the film
   4. incorrect horizontal angulation

126. The generation of x-rays requires
   1. electrons
   2. heating of the cathode
   3. a target
   4. a lead screen

127. If a patient tends to gag easily during the x-ray procedure, the assistant should
   1. allow patient to relax, then begin taking anterior films first
   2. only expose those x-rays that do not cause a gag reflex
   3. have the patient gargle with a mouth rinse
   4. place cotton rolls on either side of the film to prevent discomfort

128. When seating the patient for a radiograph, the operator should
   1. tell the patient what is being done
   2. have the patient remove eyeglasses
   3. have the patient remove partials and dentures
   4. drape the patient with a lead apron

129. Quality assurance is necessary to ensure that
   1. x-ray film is not outdated
   2. x-ray units are operating properly
   3. temperatures are accurate for processing
   4. test film runs are conducted periodically

130. Exposure time is determined by
1. kVp and mA
2. vertical angulation
3. film speed
4. horizontal angulation

131. Radiographs taken of a pregnant patient must
1. be done as quickly as possible to avoid extra exposure
2. be done with two lead lap aprons in place
3. never be done
4. be done only under a doctor's direct order in emergency situations

132. During x-ray exposure and processing procedures, appropriate infection control measures include
1. use of barrier techniques for equipment and control switches
2. use of disposable gloves
3. use of sterile film holders
4. proper disposal of contaminated gloves and outer film packet cover before day loader processing

133. Before exposing a panoramic radiograph on a patient, the dental assistant should request the removal of
1. dentures
2. eyeglasses
3. removable appliances
4. earrings

134. If x-ray films appear brownish after several months of storage, this is probably due to
1. too much sunlight in the office
2. improper fixing techniques
3. coffee stains
4. insufficient time in the wash

135. Which of the following is (are) true of extraoral films?
1. They are used when large areas of the facial structures need to be radiographed
2. They may be loaded into cassettes
3. They often are used when fractures of the mandible are suspected
4. They may be used in conjunction with intensifying screens

136. Which of the following should be present in a diagnostically acceptable panoramic radiograph?
1. The inferior border of the mandible is visible on both right and left sides of film
2. There is no incisal overlap of anterior teeth
3. The patient is symmetrically aligned so that condyles are equal distances from the top of film
4. There is uniform density with no contrast

137. Which of the following statements concerning automatic film processing units is (are) true?
1. The completely processed film can be obtained in about 5 min.
2. The same chemicals can be used as for manual processing
3. They provide standardization of development
4. They do not need to be cleaned

138. Which of the following should be performed to control manual x-ray processing solutions properly?
1. Change solutions daily
2. Cover the tank when not in use
3. Stir solutions weekly
4. Adhere to time and temperature charts of processing solutions

139. Some of the somatic effects of long-term exposure to ionizing radiation include
1. genetic deformities
2. erythema
3. alopecia
4. blood dyscrasias

140. Which of the following could the dental assistant do when exposing radiographs of an edentulous patient who has a gagging problem?
1. Expose bite-wing radiographs
2. Use a panoramic radiograph
3. Use the bisecting angle technique because the film can be placed higher in the palate or deeper in the mandibular arch
4. Use an occlusal film for each arch

141. Which of the following controls on an x-ray unit should be checked before usage?
1. Milliamperage (mA)
2. Kilovoltage potential (kVp)
3. On/off switch
4. Timer

DIRECTIONS (Questions 142–150): Each of the questions or incomplete statements in this section is followed by four suggested answers or completions. Select the **ONE** lettered answer or completion that is **BEST** in each case.

---

142. Which type of film exposure is most helpful in location of a stone or calculus accumulation in Wharton's duct?
A. Lateral jaw film
B. Periapical film
C. Tomograph
D. Occlusal film

143. What is the name of the device used to stabilize the patient's head during special extraoral exposures?
A. Laminagraph
B. Cephalostat
C. Antropometer
D. Facebow

144. A panoramic film shows a blurred area in the center that was caused by the shifting of the chair. Which type of panoramic machine was used to make the exposure?
A. Orthopantomagraphy
B. Panelipse
C. Orthoceph
D. Panorex

145. The film size for a panoramic survey is
A. $8'' \times 10''$
B. $5'' \times 10''$
C. $5'' \times 12''$
D. $8'' \times 12''$

146. The film must be placed between the intensifying screens
    A. with the blue side of the screen inside (with the film between)
    B. with the white side of the screen inside (with the film between)
    C. either side will produce acceptable results
    D. no intensifying screen is needed to produce readable radiographs

147. Film used in extraoral radiography includes
    A. intensifying screen film
    B. double-coated film
    C. screen or nonscreen film
    D. opalescent film

148. Which of the following statements is true when loading the film into the cassette before exposure (in extraoral radiography)?
    A. The film comes preloaded in the cassette
    B. The procedure must be done in the darkroom
    C. The film may be placed in the holder outside the darkroom
    D. The film does not need an intensifying screen

149. The advantages of panographic radiography are all of the following **EXCEPT**
    A. makes film exposure easier for patient
    B. eliminates the need for bite-wing x-rays
    C. saves processing and mounting time
    D. makes location of large pathologic conditions more readily identifiable

150. What type of exposure is needed to diagnose the TMJ area?
    A. Cephalometric
    B. Occlusal
    C. Panographic
    D. Lateral jaw survey

Practice Test Questions 2: Dental Radiology

Answers and Discussion

1. **(C)** The duties that can be performed legally by an assistant are determined by the Dental Practice Act of each state. It is the responsibility of the dental assistant to be aware of legal constraints.

2. **(D)** Reproductive cells are the most radiosensitive cells listed. Cells that undergo active division are the most radiosensitive. Cells ranked according to their radiosensitivity are sperm and ova, blood cells, epithelial cells, connective tissue cells, nerve cells, and muscle cells.

3. **(B)** The most penetrating x-rays have short wavelengths and high frequencies. They are called hard x-rays.

4. **(A)** Before seating the dental patient it is necessary to cover the x-ray exposure control panel with disposable plastic wrap. The plastic barrier wrap should be replaced between patients.

5. **(C)** An exposed x-ray film has been placed inside a patient's mouth and is considered contaminated.

6. **(D)** The milliamperage controls the heating of the cathode and thereby the density of the resultant electron cloud. Increasing the milliamperage will result in a denser cloud and an increase in the number of x-rays produced.

7. **(B)** If handling contaminated exposed x-ray film the dental assistant must wear gloves.

8. **(C)** The lead diaphragm determines the size and shape of the x-ray beam as it leaves the x-ray head. The distance between the target and the film will determine the size of the beam at the film.

9. **(A)** The portion of the target struck by the electrons is called the focal spot. Heat produced when electrons strike the focal spot must be dissipated, or the x-ray tube might become damaged.

10. **(D)** Proper collimation of the primary beam results in a beam that closely approximates the size and shape of the film. This decreases the patient's exposure to radiation.

11. **(A)** The kVp determines the penetrating power of the x-ray beam. Increasing the kVp increases the electrical potential between the cathode and anode. This increases the force driving the electrons from the cathode to the anode, which results in an increase in the penetrating power of the resulting x-ray beam. Dental radiology uses 45 kVp to 95 kVp.

12. **(B)** The x-ray at the center of the primary beam is called the central ray.

13. **(D)** A stepwedge may be utilized to test for quality control during manual processing procedures.

14. **(B)** Filtration is the passing of the x-ray beam through an aluminum disc to eliminate the longer, weaker wavelength x-rays. Longer wavelength x-rays, also known as soft x-rays, do not have penetrating power and could be absorbed by the patient's cheek.

15. **(C)** Material safety data sheets provide detailed information regarding a product's hazardous ingredients, including information on physical and chemical characteristics, health hazards, reactivity data, protection information, first-aid procedures, handling, storage, and waste disposal. The name and address of the manufacturer are also included.

16. (A) Scatter radiation is a type of secondary radiation created when the primary beam passes through an object.

17. (B) The penetrating power of primary radiation is greater than the penetrating power of the resulting secondary radiation produced. When the primary beam strikes an object, it gives up some energy, and the resultant secondary radiation has less energy and less penetrating power.

18. (B) X-ray processing tanks or automatic processors containing x-ray processing solutions must be labeled with the manufacturer's information as stated on the original label.

19. (C) The latent period is the time period between the effects of cumulative radiation and visible tissue damage. Some severe reactions to radiation exposure may occur in a few days. Other side effects may not appear for 20 years or more.

20. (C) The amount of radiation a person receives is cumulative in the entire body. Therefore, people working with x-rays should take proper precautions to decrease their exposure.

21. (A) Maximum protection of the patient requires that the x-rays pass through a shielded open-ended cone. X-rays passing through a closed-ended cone produce scatter radiation.

22. (B) An easy way to tell the amount of radiation one is receiving is to wear a radiation film badge. The badge is worn for a period of time, after which the radiation exposure can be measured. If the occupational dose is too high, measures must be taken to correct the problem.

23. (A) The maximum whole-body dose considered permissible is 0.1 rem/week (100 mR/week). Ideally, the operator should receive zero occupational radiation.

24. (A) In order to be protected from secondary radiation, the operator should stand at least 6′ away from the x-ray head when exposing film.

25. (B) To prevent gonadal exposure to x-rays, the patient should wear a lead apron. X-rays will not pass through lead. Therefore, the gonadal tissue, which is very sensitive to radiation, will be protected.

26. (C) If not in use, the leaded apron must be stored unfolded, preferably over a support rod. Repeated folding of the lead apron and collar will damage the material.

27. (B) The best technique to decrease radiation exposure is to use the fastest film possible.

28. (C) Film speed is determined by the size of the silver bromide crystals. Larger crystals produce faster film. Faster film requires less total radiation for exposure. Film speed ranges from A to F. D and F are the fastest.

29. (A) The radiographic film is a cellulose acetate base thinly covered on both sides with a gelatin emulsion of silver bromide salts.

30. (D) The button or dot is used to orient the films when mounting. All films should be oriented with the button in the same direction when mounting.

31. (B) The purpose of the lead foil in dental film is to prevent fogging or a darkening of the film, which may be caused from secondary radiation.

32. (C) Bite-wing films are used for diagnosis of interproximal caries, visualizing the height of interproximal bone, and determining the proximal adaptation of restorations.

33. (A) Water's film is an extraoral film used to help visualize the sinus. Extraoral films are large films that are positioned beside the patient's face. They are used to visualize large portions of the skull, mandible, or maxilla.

34. (D) X-ray films should be kept by the dentist indefinitely. The x-ray films are the property of the dentist and are part of the patient's permanent record. X-ray films may be used as evidence in a court of law.

35. (A) A lead container is recommended for storage of unexposed x-ray film to protect the film from scatter radiation. The container should also be protected from light and moisture.

36. (D) Periapical films are used to show the entire tooth and the supporting structures. They come in three sizes: small for children, regular for adults, and narrow for anterior teeth.

37. (B) The principle used in panoramic radiography is laminagraphy. Laminagraphy is the focusing of the x-ray beam at a point that will appear on the resulting film. Other objects in the beam's path are out of focus and do not appear on the radiograph.

38. (C) Radiolucency depends on the density of an object. The less dense an object, the more radiolucent it is, and the darker it will appear on radiographs.

39. (B) Radiopaque structures appear white. The denser a structure, the more radiopaque it will appear. The most radiopaque structure of a tooth is the enamel.

40. (C) The pulp chamber is radiolucent and appears dark on an x-ray.

41. (A) Caries appears radiolucent on an x-ray. Calculus, tori, and root tips are denser structures and appear radiopaque.

42. (D) The diagonal radiopaque line that is visible on the lower part of the roots of the mandibular molars is the internal oblique line.

43. (B) The small circular radiolucency near the roots of the mandibular premolars is called the mental foramen.

44. (C) The u-shaped radiopaque structure often seen in the maxillary molar area is the zygoma.

45. (B) The thin radiopaque band between the maxillary incisors is called the nasal septum.

46. (D) The heavily radiopaque midpoint of the mandible is called the symphysis.

47. (B) The small circular radiolucency below the mandibular incisor roots is called the lingual foramen.

48. (A) The large radiolucent area shown above the maxillary molar and appearing as a white line is called the maxillary sinus.

49. (D) The mandibular canal appears long, narrow, and radiolucent below the roots of the mandibular molars.

50. (A) The radiopaque circular area below the apices of the mandibular incisors is called the genial tubercles.

51. (C) The bisecting the angle technique requires that the central ray be perpendicular to the line bisecting the angle formed by the film and the tooth.

52. (B) The paralleling technique requires that the film be parallel to the tooth and that a 16″ cone be used. The central ray is directed perpendicularly to the tooth and film. The paralleling technique does not use the 8″ short cone.

53. (A) The sagittal plane of the patient's head should be perpendicular to the floor. The vertical angulation on the x-ray head is based on this position.

54. (D) The ala-tragus line is parallel to the floor when taking maxillary periapical films, bite-wing films, and maxillary occlusal films.

55. (B) When positioning the patient, the occlusal plane of the arch being radiographed should be parallel to the floor.

56. (B) Vertical angulation may be altered from patient to patient depending on anatomic structural differences, such as the height of the vault of the palate.

57. (A) The periapical films are extended 1/8″ beyond the occlusal surface or incisal edge. The resulting film should also show 3 mm beyond the root apex.

58. (C) Firm placement of the film will help prevent gagging by avoiding movement of the film over gag-sensitive areas of the palate.

59. (C) The latent image is not truly an image but a potential image composed of energized silver halide crystals. The latent image will become a visible image after processing the exposed film.

60. (A) Cone cutting is caused by the central ray not being aimed at the center of the film. This results in part of the film not being exposed to radiation.

61. (D) Black lines across the film are indicative of excessive bending that has cracked the emulsion.

62. (B) A blurred film will result if the patient moves while dental film is being exposed.

63. (D) If a patient is reluctant to be radiographed, the assistant should explain the procedure thoroughly before taking the radiographs. Emphasis on the use of safety devices, such as the lead apron and thyroid collar, to protect the body from unnecessary scatter radiation, the use of fast film to limit exposure time, and the low dosage of x-rays emitted for dental films may be presented. The doctor depends on the dental x-rays for thorough treatment planning and diagnosis.

64. (A) Less time is necessary for radiograph exposures on children because the tissues the radiation must pass through are not as dense as those of adults.

65. (B) Intensifying screens decrease exposure time of extraoral radiographs by creating an illuminating pattern of the object through which the x-ray has passed. The illuminating pattern continues to expose the film after the radiation exposure has stopped.

66. (C) As the target–film distance increases, there is less distortion because the x-rays are more parallel as they strike the object and film. If the target–film distance is increased, the exposure time must be increased to obtain a properly exposed film.

67. (C) To prevent distortion of panorex films, the patient's chin must be properly placed in the chin rest so that the head is positioned symmetrically.

68. (B) The full mouth series of a dentulous person is composed of 18–20 films. An 18-film series would consist of films of the max-

illary and mandibular central and lateral incisors, right and left canines, right and left premolars, right and left molars, and bite-
wings of the right and left premolars and right and left molars.

69. (A) Devices used to hold the film in the paralleling technique include a film holder and hemostats.

70. (D) Extraoral films are more light-sensitive than are intraoral
films.

71. (B) Increasing the mA increases the electron density and subse-
quently the quantity of the resulting x-rays. An increase in the
quantity of x-rays will result in more x-rays affecting the film and
consequently darker film.

72. (A) Elongation can be caused by insufficient vertical angulation, improper positioning of the patient's head, or improper film
placement.

73. (B) Foreshortening can be caused by too much vertical angulation, improper positioning of the patient's head, or improper film
placement.

74. (D) A herringbone pattern results if the film is exposed when it
is reversed in the patient's mouth. This pattern is caused by the radiation passing through the lead foil, which has this pattern. The
resultant film is light and cannot be used for diagnostic purposes.

75. (D) When the target–film distance is doubled, the exposure time
must be increased fourfold to maintain equal film density. This is
an example of the inverse-square law of radiation, which states
that radiation intensity is inversely proportional to the square of
the distances.

76. (A) The term density is used to describe the blackness of an exposed radiograph. An overexposed film will appear very dark
(high density), and an underexposed film will reveal much light-
ness (low density).

77. (B) The difference in density of various regions of a radiograph is called contrast. Contrast refers to how the dark and

light areas of a film are differentiated. Definition refers to the sharpness or clarity of the images outlined on the film.

78. **(A)** For maximum penetration of x-rays, a higher kVp is selected. When the kVp is increased, the x-ray wavelength is shortened and the x-ray beam emits a higher energy source (photons), allowing effective penetration of thicker structures with greater density. In order to maintain proper radiographic contrast and density, the mA must be reduced whenever the kVp is increased.

79. **(D)** Appropriate infection control procedures during x-ray exposure include the placement of a disposable plastic wrap over the x-ray tube head. The assistant should use protective barriers.

80. **(A)** Radiographs of edentulous areas should be exposed routinely to check for any pathologic conditions in the area (e.g., retained root tips, foreign bodies).

81. **(C)** Films cannot be overfixed and can be left in the fixer indefinitely.

82. **(D)** It is safe to expose radiographs to light after they have been placed in the fixer. The radiographs can be read at this time and then placed back into the fixer to complete the processing.

83. **(B)** Film fog appears as a dull gray finish on the processed film. Some causes are light leak in the darkroom, old film, or exposure of film to secondary or stray radiation.

84. **(C)** The film is washed after it is removed from the developer and before it is put in the fixer in order to wash off the developing solution and stop the developing process. Washing also removes all chemicals from the film so the fixing solution is not contaminated.

85. **(A)** The fixing solution is acidic. The following chemicals make up the fixer: sodium thiosulfate, which dissolves undeveloped silver salts; alum to shrink and harden the gelatin emulsion; sodium sulfate, a preservative against oxidation; acetic acid to increase action of the preservative; and distilled water, the medium in which the chemical activity takes place.

86. **(B)** Higher temperature will cause an increase in precipitation of the silver halide, resulting in a darker film.

87. **(D)** When a film is placed in the fixing solution unaffected (or unprecipitated), silver bromide crystals are removed. Therefore, the emulsion of an unexposed film will be removed completely, and the film will be clear.

88. **(A)** Fixing the film removes the unaffected silver halides. Areas in which these halides are removed will appear lighter in the final film. Fixing also rehardens the emulsion.

89. **(C)** The temperature of the processing solution usually is adjusted by immersing containers of the processing solution in a temperature-adjustable waterbath.

90. **(D)** Processed films left in the water overnight will lose all of their image and appear clear. Films should never be left in the water overnight.

91. **(C)** After fixing, the film is washed for 20–30 min. and then dried. If the films are washed for too long, they will become lighter because some of the precipitated silver bromide will wash off. If the films are not washed for long enough, some residue from the fixer may remain, and the films will have a brown tint.

92. **(C)** In order to develop films, the developing solution must have a basic pH. The following chemicals make up the developer: hydroquinone, an oxidizing agent that gives the film contrast; Elon, another oxidizing agent to give the film detail; sodium sulfite, a preservative to lengthen the life of the solution; sodium carbonate to make the solution basic; potassium bromide to make the aforementioned chemicals act selectively; and distilled water, the medium in which the chemical activity takes place.

93. **(B)** White spots may appear on a processed film if contaminated with fixing solution before the developing phase of processing. The silver halide crystals are unable to react with the developing solution properly, causing a whitened area to appear on the processed film.

94. (A) Reticulation is the cracking of the film emulsion due to large temperature differences between the processing solutions.

95. (D) The processed films should be dried by suspending them in air. A fan may be used to speed up the drying process. However, the films should not be allowed to touch each other or anything else until they are dry.

96. (C) Film not fixed for a long enough period of time (about 10 min.) will have a brown tint. Radiographs may be read after a short period of fixing (wet reading) but must be returned to the fixing solution to ensure complete removal of the unaffected silver bromide crystals.

97. (B) The chemicals used in processing solutions are dissolved in distilled water. Other types of water contain chemicals that can interfere with the proper processing of radiographs.

98. (C) The strength of the safelight in the darkroom is dependent on the sensitivity of the film. The faster the film, the more light-sensitive the film and, therefore, the less the strength of the safelight permitted.

99. (B) The processing solutions should be changed at least every 3–4 weeks, depending on usage. The solutions lose strength through exposure to air, heavy usage, and contamination. Regular quality assurance film test runs should be conducted to ensure that processing solutions are effective.

100. (B) The optimum time–temperature relationship for processing films varies with the manufacturer's specifications. An accepted time–temperature range is 68° F for $4\frac{1}{2}$ min.

101. (B)

102. (C)

103. (C)

104. (D)

105. (B)

106. (A)

107. (B)

108. (D)

109. (C)

110. (B)

111. (A)

112. (D)

113. (E)

114. (C)

115. (C)

116. (A)

117. (C)

118. (C)

119. (E) Extraoral films are used to help visualize fractures, pathologic conditions of the sinus, the temporomandibular joint, the position of impacted teeth, and large pathologic lesions. They are used also when a patient cannot open his or her mouth.

120. (D) The coronoid process appears radiopaque in the lower distal portion of a maxillary molar film.

121. (E) Occupational safety measures for the dental assistant operating radiographic equipment include never holding the x-ray film in the patient's mouth during exposure, always working in a shielded area (lead-lined), standing behind protective shielded areas at least 6′ away from the target area, and regular monitoring of an x-ray film badge.

122. (A) To protect the patient from unnecessary x-ray exposure, the dental assistant should drape the patient with a lead-lined apron, use technique factors that avoid retakes resulting in low patient exposure, and use fast films and x-ray machines with collimators.

123. (C) Dark films can result from overexposure (too much radiation contacts the film because of an increase in the quantity of radiation or the exposure time) or overdevelopment (more silver halide crystals are precipitated if the developing solution is too warm or if the films are left in the solution too long).

124. (B) Light films may result from underexposing (not enough radiation reaches the film because of insufficient quantity or insufficient exposure), underdeveloping (insufficient amounts of affected silver halide are precipitated; this can be caused by a cold developing solution or keeping the films in the developing solution for too short a period of time), or overwashing, resulting in lighter films because affected silver halide crystals will be washed off.

125. (D) Overlapping occurs if the central ray is not parallel to the proximal contacts in the horizontal plane. If overlapping occurs, parts of adjacent teeth are superimposed on each other, and the films cannot be used diagnostically.

126. (A) The sequence of events that leads to x-ray generation is first heating the cathode to produce an electron cloud. The density of the cloud produced depends on the milliampere (mA). Second is the creation of an electric potential between the cathode and anode (target). The speed of the crossing depends on the kilovolt (kVp). Third, the collision of the electrons with the anode produces x-rays (photons).

127. (B) If a patient tends to gag easily during the x-ray procedure, the auxiliary should allow the patient to relax, then begin taking anterior films first. The patient may also be allowed to gargle with mouthwash to help alleviate a gag reflex.

128. (E) When seating the patient for a radiograph, the operator should explain the procedure to the patient and then ask the patient to remove any prosthetic appliances, such as partials or dentures. Eyeglasses may be removed as well. Drape the patient with a lead-lined apron and thyroid lead collar.

129. (E) Methods of ensuring high-quality x-ray film exposures with minimum radiation exposure for patient and operator include instruments of quality assurance, such as regular monitoring and testing of equipment to prevent malfunctions; regular maintenance of processing solutions, including regulation of solution temperatures; and regular test film runs.

130. (B) The exposure time is determined by the mA, the kVp, the density of the bone and structures the primary beam must pass through, the film speed, and the focal (target) film distance.

131. (D) Radiographs taken of a pregnant patient must be kept at a minimum and performed only in emergency situations under the doctor's direct order.

132. (E) Infection control measures must be employed during radiographic procedures. They include protective barriers for the operator and appropriate sterilization and disinfection of equipment and x-ray armamentarium. Special procedures are followed to prevent contamination of day loader processing units. When developing films, contaminated film packets must be disposed of properly and kept from contaminating other surfaces and objects by isolating them in a separate paper cup.

133. (E) Before exposing a panoramic radiograph on a patient, the assistant should ask the patient to remove any partials or dentures, eyeglasses, and earrings.

134. (C) X-ray films may appear brownish in color due to improper fixing techniques and insufficient time in the wash. Other causes may include weak fixing solutions and outdated film.

135. (E) Extraoral radiographs are taken when the area of concern cannot be diagnosed adequately with intraoral radiographic techniques. They are used when large areas of the facial structures need to be radiographed. Situations requiring extraoral radiographs may include the use of cassettes and intensifying screens, as in panoramic radiography. Extraoral exposures allow the clinician to view impacted teeth, sinuses, cysts, jaw fractures, occlusal relationships, and lateral projections of the TMJ area.

136. (A) A diagnostically acceptable panoramic radiograph displays both right and left sides of the inferior border of the mandible and reveals no excessive overlapping of the teeth. If the patient is symmetrically aligned, the right and left condyles will be exposed at equal distances from the top of the film.

137. (B) Automatic film processing units require special types of chemical solutions unlike the manual processing tanks. The automatic processing units must be cleaned periodically and monitored to maintain optimum processed film quality. The automatic processor units provide rapid development of the exposed film and standardization of development.

138. (C) Quality control of processing solutions is necessary to ensure consistent quality of film processing techniques. When not in use, processing tanks must be covered to prevent dehydration or contamination. Time and temperature charts for processing solutions must be followed strictly during manual processing procedures. A thermometer should be available in the wash tank and checked before developing exposed x-ray film.

139. (E) Long-term effects of overexposure to ionizing radiation may cause necrotic reactions to living cells. Dangers of overexposure include cancer, blood dyscrasia, alopecia (hair loss), erythema, and genetic deformities.

140. (C) For patients with a high gag reflex, the assistant may have to take a panoramic x-ray or an occlusal film.

141. (E) Daily and weekly monitoring of x-ray equipment is necessary for quality assurance. Before use, all control devices, such as the timer, mA and kVp settings, and on/off switch, should be inspected.

142. (D) The occlusal exposure is beneficial in locating a salivary duct stone, or calculus, accumulation along the floor of the mouth. The occlusal intraoral x-ray allows for a broader view of the entire arch.

143. (B) The cephalostat is used to stabilize the patient's head during special extraoral exposures. The cephalostat holds the patient's head parallel and at right angles to the x-ray beam.

144. (D) The panorex machine requires movement of the chair to complete the film exposure of the other half of the x-ray film, resulting in a white unexposed strip extending vertically down the center of the exposed film. The panorex extraoral radiograph shows the complete maxillary and mandibular arch in one exposure.

145. (C) The film size for a panoramic survey is 5" × 12".

146. (B) The unexposed film is placed at the base of the opened intensifying screen. The white side of the intensifying screen must be on the inside, with the film in between. The intensifying screen allows production of a film with greater diagnostic quality through a minimum amount of radiation.

147. (C) Screen and nonscreen film is used for extraoral radiographs. Screen film is designed to be used in a cassette holder with an intensifying screen, and nonscreen film is designed for use in a cardboard exposure holder.

148. (B) When loading extraoral film into the cassette, the procedure must always be done in the darkroom, since the x-ray film is light sensitive.

149. (B) Panoramic radiography does not eliminate the need for bite-wing x-rays because the panoramic x-ray is an extraoral film. It is exposed outside the patient's mouth, and there is loss of detail in the radiograph. Interproximal caries can best be detected by intraoral bite-wing film exposures.

150. (D) The lateral jaw survey is used to diagnose the TMJ area. A 5" × 7" film is used and placed extraorally along the mandible and centered over the first molars.

Practice Test Questions 3: Infection Control

DIRECTIONS (Questions 1–15): Each of the questions or incomplete statements in this section is followed by four suggested answers or completions. Select the ONE lettered answer or completion that is BEST in each case.

1. Which are the smallest microbes?
    A. Viruses
    B. Fungi
    C. Bacteria
    D. Algae

2. Bactericidal refers to
    A. inhibiting bacterial growth
    B. bacteria in the bloodstream
    C. killing bacteria
    D. the effect of bacteria on people

3. What becomes contaminated in the operatory with each operation?
    A. Dental charts
    B. Reception area
    C. Floor
    D. All surfaces that come in contact with any microbes from the patient's mouth

4. A protective nongrowing form of a microorganism is referred to as a
   A. spore
   B. fungus
   C. cell
   D. virus

5. The ultrasonic cleaner is used to
   A. sterilize handpieces
   B. clean instruments
   C. sterilize instruments
   D. pasteurize fluids

6. Instruments are washed before being autoclaved
   A. to prevent rusting
   B. to prevent debris from harboring microbes
   C. to kill any spores
   D. to kill any viruses

7. A surgical mask is used during a dental operation to
   A. avoid odors of various dental materials
   B. protect the patient from inhaling the aerosol created by the high-speed handpiece
   C. protect the operator and assistant from inhaling the aerosol created by the high-speed handpiece
   D. protect the patient from inhaling the aerosol created by the low-speed handpiece

8. Carbon steel instruments are best sterilized by
   A. dry heat
   B. autoclaving
   C. disinfectants
   D. flaming

9. The most effective way to kill microbes is
   A. cold sterilization
   B. boiling water
   C. autoclaving
   D. ultraviolet light

10. How can you tell whether a package of instruments has been autoclaved?
    A. Temperature-sensitive tape will turn color
    B. Instruments are a different color after being autoclaved
    C. The autoclave bags are left open
    D. Instruments feel warm

11. The effectiveness of a disinfectant solution is altered by the
    A. number of instruments
    B. dilution with water
    C. room temperature
    D. number of bacteria on the instruments

12. A person who harbors a disease without feeling its effect is called a
    A. retainer
    B. transmitter
    C. carrier
    D. neophyte

13. The passage of an infectious microbe from one patient to another is called
    A. plague
    B. rehosting
    C. microbe transfer
    D. cross-infection

14. Dental laboratory infection control includes disinfection of all of the following EXCEPT
    A. rubber bite blocks
    B. impressions
    C. gypsum casts
    D. wax registration records

15. Dental prostheses should be disinfected
    A. with soap and water
    B. daily with an immersion agent
    C. before sending to the laboratory
    D. never disinfect a dental prosthesis

DIRECTIONS (Questions 16–23): For each of the items in this section, **ONE** or **MORE** of the numbered options is correct. Choose answer
- **A.** if only 1, 2, and 3 are correct
- **B.** if only 1 and 3 are correct
- **C.** if only 2 and 4 are correct
- **D.** if only 4 is correct
- **E.** if all are correct

16. Hands should be washed
    1. before and after using gloves
    2. with an antimicrobial soap
    3. for a full 15 sec. between each patient
    4. for a full 5 min. if part of a surgical dental team

17. The term universal precautions implies that
    1. every patient must complete a medical history before treatment
    2. all patients are apprehensive
    3. gloves and face masks should be used when treating infectious patients only
    4. infection control procedures should be implemented for all patients

18. Protective barriers for the dental staff may include
    1. disposable gowns
    2. protective eyewear/face shield
    3. disposable gloves and face mask
    4. lead-lined aprons

19. Chairside infection control includes the use of
    1. a high-velocity evacuation system
    2. preset trays
    3. rubber dam whenever possible
    4. proper waste disposal methods

20. Radiographic infection control includes
    1. use of barriers for x-ray equipment
    2. using sterilized film
    3. placing exposed films in isolation paper cups
    4. changing processing solutions weekly

21. Dental handpieces should be
    1. autoclaved after each use
    2. oiled weekly with sterile solutions
    3. disinfected only with an approved disinfectant spray
    4. sterilized according to manufacturer's directions

22. Disposal of infectious waste includes
    1. the use of sturdy leakproof bags
    2. labeling bags as hazardous waste
    3. disposing according to state and local regulations
    4. a sealed, puncture-resistant container for needles, blades, and broken glass

23. If performing CPR on a patient with a history of an infectious disease, the rescuer should always
    1. wear disposable gloves
    2. not perform CPR until medical assistance arrives
    3. use protective devices or a microshield
    4. obtain a thorough health history first before beginning CPR

DIRECTIONS (Questions 24–44): Each of the questions or incomplete statements in this section is followed by four suggested answers or completions. Selection the **ONE** lettered answer or completion that is **BEST** in each case.

---

24. Which of the following statements is **NOT** true about gloves?
    A. Gloves must be worn at all times when the operator is in contact with blood, saliva, and mucous
    B. Gloves should be changed for each patient
    C. Handwashing is not necessary when you are wearing gloves
    D. A heavier glove that is puncture resistant should be utilized when handling soiled instruments for sterilization preparation

25. Following each use, the nitrous oxide rubber tubing and mask must be
    A. disinfected only
    B. sterilized
    C. washed with soap and hot water only
    D. thrown away

26. An oral fungal infection is called
    A. leukoplakia
    B. thrush/candidiasis
    C. herpes
    D. nevi

27. White patches on the soft tissues are called
    A. leukoplakia
    B. Fordyce's granules
    C. tori
    D. fibromas

28. Erythema is
    A. a type of oral carcinoma
    B. cryotherapy
    C. redness of the skin
    D. a form of bacteria

29. Immunology refers to the study of
    A. resistance to disease
    B. factors that cause disease
    C. population studies
    D. fluoridation

30. Which of these terms describes cracks or peeling at the angle of the mouth?
    A. Cellulitis
    B. Cheilosis
    C. Keratosis
    D. Exostosis

31. The ability to ward off disease is known as
    A. infection
    B. host resistance
    C. postponement
    D. the autogenic ability

32. An antibody is
    A. an autoimmune disease
    B. part of the body's defense system

C. an enzyme
D. a catalyst

33. Bacterial invasion of the circulatory system is referred to as
 A. hyperemia
 B. toxemia
 C. bacteremia
 D. granuloma

34. A recurrent viral infection in the mouth is
 A. pyogenic granuloma
 B. herpes simplex
 C. aphthous ulcer
 D. thrush

35. Acute necrotizing ulcerative gingivitis often is referred to as
 A. trench mouth
 B. pregnancy tumor
 C. gingivosis
 D. epulis

36. HIV/AIDS is a disease of
 A. the endocrine system
 B. the immune system
 C. the oral cavity
 D. noninfectious origins

37. The major mode of transmission for HIV is
 A. sweat
 B. tears
 C. urine
 D. contact with contaminated blood

38. Surgical blades and contaminated needles should be disposed of in
 a (an)
 A. sealed metal container
 B. sealed plastic bag
 C. sharps puncture-proof container
 D. open trash container with biohazard symbol

39. Heavy-duty utility gloves must be worn when
   A. taking x-rays
   B. preparing sterile instrument trays
   C. decontaminating a dental operatory
   D. assisting in surgical procedures

40. Environmental surface disinfectants may include
   A. hydrogen peroxide
   B. EPA-approved chemical disinfectants
   C. ethyl alcohol
   D. quaternary ammonium compounds

41. Approved methods of sterilization include all of the following **EXCEPT**
   A. alcohol immersion
   B. dry heat
   C. ethylene oxide gas
   D. chemical vapor

42. Routine monitoring of sterilization cycles can best be accomplished by utilizing
   A. heat sensitive tape
   B. heat sensitive autoclave instrument bags
   C. biological spore tests
   D. readings on the pressure dials

43. Instruments that are classified as "critical" or "semicritical" must be
   A. disinfected
   B. sterilized
   C. immersed in an ultrasonic cleaning solution
   D. hand-scrubbed with an antimicrobial soap

44. Following OSHA guidelines if an employee refuses to obtain the hepatitis vaccination the employer is required to
   A. dismiss the employee
   B. ask the employee not to participate in surgical procedures
   C. have the employee sign an informed refusal/declination form
   D. have the employee double glove for all procedures

DIRECTIONS (Questions 45–54): Match the term in Column A with the description in Column B.

COLUMN A

45. Sodium
    hypochlorite _____
46. Synthetic phenols _____
47. Glutaraldehyde _____
48. Quaternary
    ammonium
    compounds _____
49. Isopropyl alcohol _____

COLUMN B

A. EPA registered as suitable
   chemical sterilant
B. used for preparation of the
   skin prior to injection
C. EPA registered as suitable
   surface disinfectant
D. non-tuberculocidal, serves as
   cleaning agent
E. household bleach

COLUMN A

50. sterilization _____
51. asepsis _____
52. decontamination _____
53. disinfectant _____
54. bioburden _____

COLUMN B

A. chemical agent that kills organisms but not bacterial
   spores
B. microbial or organic material
   on an object prior to decontamination
C. process by which all forms of
   organisms are destroyed by
   physical or chemical means
D. use of physical or chemical
   means to remove pathogens or
   bioburden
E. free from contamination, a
   sterile environment

DIRECTIONS (Questions 55–61): Each of the questions or incomplete statements in this section is followed by four suggested answers or completions. Selection the **ONE** lettered answer or completion that is **BEST** in each case.

55. The proper sequence used to prepare dental instruments that have penetrated soft tissue or bone ("category critical") for sterilization is
    A. disinfect, rinse, dry, oil, package, sterilize, unwrap
    B. preclean, disinfect with low-level chemicals, rinse, dry, package
    C. preclean, rinse, dry, package, sterilize, store package
    D. disinfect in ultrasonic unit with high-level EPA approved chemicals, rinse, dry, store in instrument drawer

56. Before sending an impression to the laboratory technician it is necessary to perform all of the following steps **EXCEPT**
    A. use protective barriers, clothing, gloves, masks, during the initial rinsing of the impression
    B. thoroughly dry the impression, then wrap for sterilization
    C. spray the impression according to the manufacturer's recommendation with an approved disinfectant
    D. isolate contaminated impressions and place in leak-proof closed container with biohazard label prior to lab transport

57. The best way to recap a needle is
    A. to utilize the one-handed scoop technique
    B. to disengage the needle from syringe, then recap
    C. to use a puncture-proof sharps container
    D. to have the dentist replace the cap using the two-handed technique

58. To effectively remove bioburden from contaminated instruments prior to sterilization
    A. submerge instruments in ultrasonic cleaning unit for 10 min.
    B. soak instruments in hot soapy water, then handscrub thoroughly
    C. wipe each instrument with a disinfectant-saturated 2 × 2 gauze square
    D. bioburden does not need to be removed prior to sterilization

59. OSHA standards regarding contaminated laundry include all of the following **EXCEPT**
A. it must be handled as little as possible
B. laundry transport bags must be labeled with a biohazard symbol
C. a washer and dryer may be used on-site
D. employee training is not required

60. A Material Safety Data Sheet (MSDS) provides information which
A. must be entered in a patient's medical history
B. describes product handling, health hazards, storage, and waste disposal
C. must be entered in an employee's personnel record
D. describes precautions for the blood-borne pathogen standard

61. The National Institute for Occupational Safety and Health (NIOSH) approved mask is required when working with
A. x-rays
B. fire extinguishers
C. gypsum materials
D. sharps

DIRECTIONS (Questions 62–68): For each of the items in this section, **ONE** or **MORE** of the numbered options is correct. Choose answer
A. if only 1, 2, and 3 are correct
B. if only 1 and 3 are correct
C. if only 2 and 4 are correct
D. if only 4 is correct
E. if all are correct

---

62. To limit the spread of potentially infectious spatter and blood-contaminated saliva it is best to
1. work with a rubber dam
2. utilize a high-velocity evacuator
3. use a splash guard when operating the lathe or rag wheel
4. place a lid over the ultrasonic unit during operation

63. When handling dentin bonding materials and methacrylate resins, which of the following precautions is (are) recommended?
   1. Avoid direct contact with skin when handling
   2. Work in a well-lighted area that is cool
   3. Work in well-ventilated areas
   4. Store in a sealed glass container labeled biohazard

64. Under OSHA guidelines which of the following is (are) considered regulated waste?
   1. Blood contaminated gauze and cotton rolls
   2. Extracted teeth and biopsy specimens
   3. Sharps, needles, and scalpels
   4. Biological monitoring indicators

65. Labeling of hazardous products in the dental office is required if the hazardous product
   1. is to be used immediately within an 8-hr. shift
   2. has an original label from the manufacturer
   3. is a prescription item
   4. is transferred to a secondary container

66. If a caustic chemical comes in contact with the eyes, which of the following steps must be taken?
   1. Close eyes and apply a wet compress to forehead
   2. Flush eyes with water and seek medical attention as quickly as possible
   3. Close eyes and apply dark tinted safety glasses
   4. An incident report documenting route of exposure must be completed

67. When working with mercury during an amalgam preparation
   1. a mask must be worn to prevent inhaling mercury vapors
   2. gloves must be worn to avoid direct skin contact
   3. the work area must be well ventilated
   4. use a mercury spill clean-up kit for accidental spills

68. OSHA guidelines require employers to establish a written exposure control plan which includes
   1. engineering and work practice controls
   2. identification of job classifications and risks

3. information on exposure incident reporting
4. employee's medical records

DIRECTIONS (Questions 69–100): Each of the questions or incomplete statements in this section is followed by four suggested answers or completions. Select the **ONE** lettered answer or completion that is **BEST** in each case.

---

69. Which of the following is required when working with white visible light-cured materials?
    A. Protective tinted visible light eyewear
    B. Safety goggles with side shields
    C. Full face shield
    D. Temperature regulated eyewash station

70. OSHA's Blood-Borne Pathogen Standard identifies dental operatory housekeeping procedures as
    A. washing windows
    B. decontaminating inanimate surfaces with approved surface disinfectant
    C. polishing dental units
    D. inventory of operatory supplies

71. If removable dentures are polished in a dental laboratory, which of the following infection control procedures must be followed?
    A. Soak dentures in mouthwash for 30 min. after polishing
    B. Place dentures in ultrasonic holding solution for 5 min.
    C. Soak dentures in mouthwash for 30 min. before polishing
    D. Remove rag polishing wheels, launder, and sterilize

72. OSHA requires that employers provide employees all of the following **EXCEPT**
    A. HBV vaccine at no charge
    B. personal protective equipment
    C. area in which to eat, drink, and smoke
    D. information and training within 10 days of employment on office written exposure control plan

73. If an immunized dental health care worker experiences a percutaneous injury from a patient who is HBsAG (hepatitis B surface antigen) negative, the exposed worker should
   A. not need further treatment once immunized
   B. start the hepatitis vaccine series immediately
   C. test for antibody to hepatitis B surface antigen
   D. request HBIG (hepatitis B immune globulin) booster

74. The assistant should review the patient's medical record for information on
   A. financial arrangements and payment history
   B. results of lab reports of antibody-antigen tests
   C. infectious diseases requiring universal precautions
   D. previous insurance malpractice claims

75. A potential health hazard for the operator while polishing contaminated appliances with motor driven or air-abrasive polishing devices arises from
   A. heat generated during polishing
   B. removal of surface fluoride
   C. contaminated aerosol produced during polishing
   D. use of highly abrasive polishing agents

76. The OSHA Hazard Communication Standard provides the employee with information regarding all of the following **EXCEPT**
   A. fire safety and clean-up procedures for acid spills
   B. ventilation requirements for chemical vapor sterilization
   C. training sessions for safe handling of hazardous chemicals including radiographic processing chemicals
   D. education regarding the benefits of vaccinations

77. Confidential employee medical records must be maintained by the employer under OSHA guidelines for the duration of employment
   A. plus 10 yr.
   B. plus 20 yr.
   C. plus 30 yr.
   D. plus 40 yr.

78. Biological indicators containing bacillus stearothermophilus spores are used to monitor
    A. steam sterilizers
    B. dry heat sterilizers
    C. ethylene oxide sterilizers
    D. high-level disinfectants

79. The microorganism associated with tuberculosis is
    A. *treponema pallidum*
    B. *neisseria gonorrhoeae*
    C. *streptococcus mutans*
    D. *mycobacterium tuberculosis*

80. Herpetic whitlow is caused by
    A. bacteria
    B. herpes simplex virus
    C. fungi
    D. hepatitis

81. A lesion associated with the primary stage of syphilis is
    A. apthous ulcer
    B. chancre
    C. herpetic whitlow
    D. gumma

82. The human immunodeficiency virus can be transmitted from all of the following **EXCEPT:**
    A. contaminated eating utensils
    B. accidental occupational exposure to blood
    C. contaminated shared tattoo needles
    D. infected mother to child during breast feeding

83. Tetanus is caused by a
    A. fungus
    B. virus
    C. spore-forming bacillus
    D. spirochete

84. The varicella-zoster virus is responsible for
   A. mumps
   B. smallpox
   C. measles
   D. chickenpox

85. After packaging instruments for sterilization the autoclave should be loaded
   A. quickly to prevent heat from escaping
   B. by placing instrument packs in an upright position
   C. without a biological indicator
   D. with as many instrument packs as possible

86. A disadvantage of the chemical vapor sterilizer is
   A. instuments become tarnished and rusted
   B. instruments must be aerated
   C. adequate ventilation is required
   D. sterilizes carbide instruments only

87. If HBsAg antibodies are present this indicates
   A. immunity
   B. active disease state
   C. natural immunity
   D. lab tests must be repeated

88. Instruments that have been sterilized but are not packaged or wrapped must be
   A. resterilized
   B. utilized immediately
   C. stored in a disinfected cabinet
   D. placed in sealed pouches as quickly as possible

89. Which of the following forms of hand cleansers is recommended for routine handwashing procedures throughout the day?
   A. Antimicrobial powdered soap
   B. Antimicrobial bar soap
   C. Alcohol wipes
   D. Antimicrobial liquid soap

90. Heat-sensitive items are sterilized by using
    A. povidone iodine
    B. alcohol
    C. high-level disinfectants
    D. intermediate level disinfectants

91. The risk of infection is increased if all of the following conditions are present **EXCEPT**
    A. protective barriers
    B. susceptible host
    C. pathogens
    D. portal of entry into body

92. In the case of sterilization failure the biologic indicator test results will be
    A. negative
    B. positive
    C. neutral
    D. without growth

93. Which type of gloves may be washed, sterilized, and reused?
    A. Utility gloves
    B. Surgical gloves
    C. Overgloves
    D. Latex gloves

94. Health care workers are at greatest risk for exposure to infection by
    A. managing waste disposal
    B. cleaning water unit lines
    C. parenteral transmission of blood-borne pathogens
    D. handling extracted teeth specimens

95. Spiral-shaped bacteria are called
    A. bacilli
    B. rickettsiae
    C. cocci
    D. spirochetes

96. A protective barrier plastic wrap is utilized on
  - **A.** disposable prophy angles
  - **B.** head of x-ray machine
  - **C.** sharps containers
  - **D.** biohazard containers

97. All of the following are true regarding the use of an ultrasonic cleaning unit **EXCEPT**
  - **A.** utilizes sound waves to cause cavitation
  - **B.** removes all forms of bioburden
  - **D.** minimizes the potential for puncture wounds
  - **D.** utilized prior to sterilization

98. To be effective, immersion of instruments in glutaraldehyde for high-level sterilization must be maintained for
  - **A.** 10 hr.
  - **B.** 30 min.
  - **C.** 1 hr.
  - **D.** 5 hr.

99. Dry heat and ethylene oxide sterilizers utilize biological indicators that contain spores of
  - **A.** *bacillus stearothermophilus*
  - **B.** *staphylococci*
  - **C.** *bacillus subtilis*
  - **D.** *treponema pallidum*

100. Labels on disinfectants must include all of the following **EXCEPT**
  - **A.** EPA number and shelf life
  - **B.** information stating tuberculocidal properties
  - **C.** preventive and first aid measures
  - **D.** ADA seal of approval

Practice Test Questions 3: Infection Control

Answers and Discussion

1. **(A)** Viruses, the smallest microbes, are composed of DNA or RNA in a protein coat. Viruses are cuboidal, spherical, elongated, or tadpole-like. Some diseases caused by viruses are herpes simplex, infectious and serum hepatitis, rabies, influenza, poliomyelitis, and AIDS.

2. **(C)** Bactericidal refers to killing bacteria. Bacteriostatic refers to inhibiting bacterial growth. Bacteremia is the presence of bacteria in the bloodstream.

3. **(D)** All surfaces in the operatory that come in contact with microbes from the patient's mouth become contaminated, including instruments, equipment, and people.

4. **(A)** Spores are a protective bacterial form. Some bacteria assume this form under unfavorable conditions. When conditions are again favorable, the bacterium will emerge from its spore form and begin to grow again.

5. **(B)** Ultrasonic cleaners can be used to debride and cleanse instruments. After removing instruments from the ultrasonic bath, rinse instruments thoroughly and dry before sterilization procedures. The ultrasonic cleaner does not sterilize instruments.

6. **(B)** Instruments must be washed thoroughly before any sterilization technique is employed. Debris not removed could harbor

bacteria and insulate them from the bactericidal effect of the sterilization technique.

7. **(C)** When using a high-speed handpiece, an aerosol is created that consists of water spray, saliva, microbes from the patient's mouth, and debris (e.g., tooth-filling material). The aerosol could cause respiratory infections to the operator and assistant. The use of a surgical mask will avoid the inhalation of the aerosol. Protective glasses will prevent eye injuries from flying debris.

8. **(A)** Carbon steel instruments are best sterilized by dry heat. This procedure will avoid rusting and dulling of sharp edges.

9. **(C)** Autoclaving, steam under pressure, is the most effective way to kill microbes. The heat from the steam sterilizes the instruments.

10. **(A)** A thermochromatic indicator tape, part of the sterilization package, will change color after it has been autoclaved.

11. **(B)** The effectiveness of a disinfectant solution is altered by dilution. Wet instruments placed in disinfectant solution will dilute the concentration. Therefore, the solution will not kill the organisms it is capable of killing in its correct concentration. Effective disinfectants should include an EPA approval number and are labeled as sterilants/disinfectants. The label states tuberculocidal, virucidal, bacteriocidal, and fungicidal properties.

12. **(C)** A person who harbors a disease without feeling its effect is a carrier. The carrier might be a person who has never had symptoms of the disease or a person recovering from the disease. A carrier can transmit the disease to other people.

13. **(D)** The passage of an infectious microbe from one patient to another is called cross-infection. This is an indirect transmission of disease and may take the following route in dentistry: patient's mouth, contaminated hand instruments, another patient's mouth.

14. **(A)** The dental laboratory can harbor numerous infectious microorganisms and assistants must follow appropriate infection control procedures to prevent disease transmission. Rubber bite blocks must be sterilized according to the manufacturer's direc-

tions either by steam autoclave or ethylene oxide methods. Impressions, wax bite registrations, and gypsum cast models (once separated from the impression) should be disinfected with an approved disinfectant agent once they have come in contact with the patient's mouth.

15. **(C)** Dental prosthesis should be disinfected before sending to the laboratory to prevent disease transmission. A dilute sodium hypochlorite solution can be used to soak and disinfect the prosthesis.

16. **(E)** Hands should be washed before placing and removing gloves with an antimicrobial soap for 10–15 sec. If part of a dental surgical team, it is necessary to perform a thorough surgical scrub for 5–10 min. on the hands, wrists, and arms up to 2″ above the elbow. Remove jewelry prior to hand washing since microorganisms can become lodged in crevices of rings and watchbands.

17. **(D)** The term universal precautions is an approach established by the Centers for Disease Control (CDC) that implies that all patients should be treated as if they were infective and advocates the use of the same infection control practices for all patients.

18. **(A)** Protective barriers for the dental staff may include disposable gowns, protective eyewear, face shields, disposable gloves, and disposable masks.

19. **(E)** Chairside infection control includes the use of a high-velocity evacuation system to reduce the amount of spatter during the use the handpiece or ultrasonic equipment. Application of a rubber dam also is recommended to minimize the spatter of blood and saliva. Preplanning needed instruments by presetting trays eliminates reaching into instrument cabinets during chairside procedures with soiled gloves. Chairside infection control also includes the use of proper waste disposal methods.

20. **(B)** Radiographic infection control measures include the use of barriers, such as a polyethylene bag over the x-ray tube head, and the placement of exposed x-ray film in isolation paper cups to prevent cross-contamination.

21. (D) Dental handpieces should be sterilized according to the manufacturer's directions. Some types of handpieces can be auto-claved (steam under pressure), but others cannot and must be disinfected with an approved agent.

22. (E) Disposal of infectious contaminated waste must be conducted according to the laws and regulations for waste disposal in each state. Standard guidelines for infectious waste disposal include the use of leakproof bags that are labeled appropriately as hazardous or infectious waste. A puncture-proof, sealed container should be used for all sharp items, such as needles, blades, disposable syringes, and broken glass.

23. (B) If performing CPR on a patient with a history of an infectious disease, the rescuer should wear disposable gloves and use a protective microshield over the victim's mouth and face.

24. (C) Washing of hands is necessary before and after wearing gloves.

25. (B) The nitrous oxide rubber tubing and mask must be sterilized after each use. Appropriate methods of sterilization must be used according to manufacturer's recommendations. Most rubber items can be sterilized safely in a gas sterilizer using ethylene oxide. Proper time and temperature for adequate sterilization and aeration after the cycle are important. Some rubber nitrous oxide nasal nose pieces are disposable. Most rubber tubing is not disposable. Before sterilization, it is best to wash the rubber nose piece with soap and water.

26. (B) Thrush, or moniliasis, is caused by the fungus *Candida albicans*. This organism is found normally in the oral cavity. An imbalance attributable to nutritional problems or antibiotic therapy is responsible for its overgrowth and the subsequent disease state.

27. (A) A white patch in the oral cavity is called leukoplakia. The cause is a chronic irritant, such as smoking or rubbing by the sharp edge of a fractured tooth. Some leukoplakia areas undergo changes and become carcinomas.

28. (C) Erythema is an abnormal redness of the skin attributable to inflammation, x-ray treatment, or a disease process.

29. **(A)** Immunology is the study of resistance to disease. Immunity can be acquired or natural. Natural immunity is obtained in utero, and acquired immunity is obtained after birth as the result of antibodies being introduced by injection or as the result of infection.

30. **(B)** Cheilosis is a condition caused by a nutritional deficiency of vitamin B (riboflavin). The condition is characterized by cracks or fissures at the angle of the mouth and a dry, cracked surface of the lips.

31. **(B)** The ability to ward off disease is known as host resistance. It can be natural, such as elements in saliva that decrease the caries rate, or acquired, such as the decrease in tooth solubility caused by the incorporation of fluoride into the tooth.

32. **(B)** Antibodies are proteins that are part of the body's defense system. They are produced in response to a foreign body, an antigen. Immunity, the ability of the body to resist infection, depends on the formation of antibodies.

33. **(C)** Bacterial invasion of the circulatory system is referred to as bacteremia. This type of infection usually involves the whole body and is known as a systemic infection.

34. **(B)** Herpes simplex is the virus that causes recurrent sores in the oral cavity. The disease is initiated by an attack of primary herpes, which is contagious in young children. The lesions of primary herpes are widespread throughout the mouth. Subsequent attacks usually are associated with single lesions. There is no known specific treatment for the lesions, which take about 14 days to heal.

35. **(A)** Another term for acute necrotizing ulcerative gingivitis (ANUG) is trench mouth or Vincent's disease. Symptoms of ANUG include ulcerations on the gingiva, bleeding gums, sloughing gingival tissues, and elevated temperature. Patients with a history of AIDS commonly exhibit gingival symptoms similar to those of ANUG.

36. **(B)** AIDS is a disease of the immune system. The acquired immunodeficiency syndrome (AIDS) is a fatal condition with a variety of symptoms that affect the entire body, including the oral cavity. AIDS is caused by the human immunodeficiency virus (HIV).

37. (D)   The major mode of transmission for HIV is through contact with contaminated blood.

38. (C)   Sharps, including needles, scalpels, and ortho arch wires, must be disposed of in a designated sharps container which is puncture-proof and leakproof and contains the biohazard symbol. The sharps container should be located as close as possible to the work area.

39. (C)   Heavy utility gloves must be utilized when decontaminating a dental operatory. The employee is also required to use other personal protective equipment during the decontamination process.

40. (B)   Environmental surface disinfectants may include EPA-registered approved chemical disinfectants. The disinfectant of choice is dependent upon the application of use, e.g., general housekeeping, intermediate-level disinfection, high-level disinfection.

41. (A)   Approved methods of sterilization do not include alcohol immersion.

42. (C)   Biological spore testing is required on a weekly basis to monitor office sterilizers.

43. (B)   Instruments that are classified as "critical" touch bone and penetrate soft tissue and must be sterilized. "Semicritical" instruments touch mucous membranes but do not penetrate soft tissue. Sterilize if possible or use high-level disinfection with semicritical instruments.

44. (C)   If an employee refuses the hepatitis B vaccination a declination form providing the employer with documentation of informed refusal is submitted by the employee.

45. (E)

46. (C)

47. (A)

48. (D)

49. (B)

50. (C)

51. (E)

52. (D)

53. (A)

54. (B)

55. (C) The appropriate sequence for preparing instruments that are categorized as critical is to preclean, rinse, dry, package, sterilize, store package. The assistant must use personal protective equipment and wear heavy utility gloves during decontanimation and instrument processing procedures.

56. (B) The impression must be disinfected according to the manufacturer's directions. Thoroughly drying and sterilizing the impression will ruin the integrity of the impression.

57. (A) The best way to prevent an accidental needle stick, occupational exposure is to utilize the one-handed scoop technique.

58. (A) Use of an ultrasonic cleaner is recommended to remove bioburden from contaminated instruments. Avoid hand scrubbing of contaminated instruments to reduce occupational exposure risks.

59. (D) Employee training is required regarding the steps for handling, transporting, and/or decontaminating soiled laundry.

60. (B) The MSDS describes product handling, health hazards, storage, waste disposal methods, and use of personal protective equipment for the employee.

61. (C) Gypsum products may irritate the eyes and impair the respiratory system. The assistant should work in an area equipped with an exhaust system and utilize personal protective equipment including a NIOSH-approved mask.

62. (E) To limit the spread of potentially infectious spatter and blood-contaminated saliva all of the listed procedures should be practiced.

63. (B) When handling dentin bonding materials and methacrylate resins avoid direct contact with the skin and work in well-ventilated areas.

64. (A) OSHA defines regulated waste as infectious materials and items that would release blood or other potentially infectious materials if compressed. Sharps, extracted teeth, and body tissues/biopsy specimens are also considered infectious or hazardous waste and must be disposed of according to state and local regulations.

65. (D) Labeling of hazardous products is required if the product is transferred to a secondary container. Labeling provides important information regarding directions for product use, disposal, storage, and personal protection requirements when handling. X-ray tanks containing developer and fixer solutions are examples of secondary containers that require labeling.

66. (C) If a caustic substance comes in contact with the eyes, flush the eyes immediately at a temperature regulated eyewash station or with fresh running water and seek medical attention as quickly as possible. The employee must report exposure incidents in the workplace to the employer.

67. (E) When working with mercury, personal protective equipment must be utilized. A well-ventilated work area and use of a commercially available mercury spill clean-up kit for accidental spills are recommended.

68. (A) Exposure control plans must include engineering and work practice controls which assist in removing the potential hazard from the employee and alter the manner in which a task is performed. Information on job classifications and identification of task risks and exposure incident reporting procedures are also required in the exposure control plan.

69. **(A)** Protective tinted visible light eyewear is required when working with white visible light-cured products.

70. **(B)** OSHA's Blood-Borne Pathogen Standard requires employers to implement a safe/sanitary work environment. Decontaminating inanimate surfaces with an EPA-approved surface disinfectant is recommended after each patient treatment procedure. Additional housekeeping OSHA recommendations include proper handling of sharps, regulated waste, broken glass, and infectious materials spills.

71. **(D)** If dentures are polished in a dental laboratory appropriate infection control procedures must be practiced including the removal of contaminated rag wheels. Rag wheels are laundered and autoclaved.

72. **(C)** OSHA does not require the employer to provide the employee with an area in which to eat, drink, and smoke. OSHA prohibits eating, drinking, smoking, application of make-up, lip balm, and handling of contact lenses in areas of the office where there is risk for occupational exposure.

73. **(A)** If a dental health care worker is immunized for hepatitis B and is exposed through a percutaneous injury to a source individual who has tested HBsAG (hepatitis B surface antigen) negative no further treatment or vaccinations are necessary for the health care worker.

74. **(B)** The patient's medical record provides information on antibody-antigen tests. The assistant should review the lab reports for information regarding immunity status and positive and negative test results. All patients should be considered to be infectious and universal precautions should be applied with all patients.

75. **(C)** A potential health hazard for the operator is inhalation of the contaminated aerosol produced during motor-driven or air-abrasive polishing. Appropriate personal protective equipment is required for the assistant.

76. **(D)** The OSHA Hazard Communication Standard provides the employee with information and training regarding the potential dangers associated with hazardous chemicals and products in the dental office. Fire safety and information on disposal and clean-up procedures for hazardous chemicals are included in this standard. The OSHA Blood-Borne Pathogen Standard protects the employee from transmission of blood-borne diseases such as HBV and HIV.

77. **(C)** Confidential employee medical records must be maintained by the employer for the duration of employment plus 30 years. The records contain information on history of hepatitis B vaccinations, exposure incidents, follow-up treatment, and postexposure evaluation, counseling, etc.

78. **(A)** Indicators containing bacillus stearothermophilus are used to monitor steam sterilizers.

79. **(D)** *Mycobacterium tuberculosis* is the organism responsible for the communicable disease tuberculosis.

80. **(B)** Herpetic whitlow is a herpetic lesion of the fingers caused by the herpes simplex virus.

81. **(B)** The chancre is a lesion associated with the primary stage of syphilis.

82. **(A)** The human immunodeficiency virus cannot be transmitted from contaminated eating utensils.

83. **(C)** Tetanus is caused by a spore-forming bacillus found in soil, dust, and animal or human feces.

84. **(D)** The varicella-zoster virus is responsible for chickenpox.

85. **(B)** Instrument packs should be loaded in the sterilizer in an upright position to allow for adequate circulation of steam and heat under pressure in the chamber.

86. **(C)** A disadvantage of the chemical vapor sterilizer is that adequate ventilation must be provided to avoid inhalation of the chemical vapor gases released by the unit.

87. (A) If HBsAg antibodies are present this indicates immunity.

88. (B) Instruments that have been sterilized but are not packaged or wrapped must be utilized immediately.

89. (D) An antimicrobial liquid soap is recommended for handwashing.

90. (C) Heat-sensitive items are sterilized by using high-level sterilant disinfectants.

91. (A) Protective barriers such as PPE for the healthcare worker assist in preventing the risk of infection. The chain of disease transmission is increased if there is a susceptible host, pathogens, and an appropriate portal of entry into the body.

92. (B) Positive test results indicate sterilization failure and retesting should be performed. Do not utilize the sterilizer until the problem has been identified and corrected.

93. (A) Utility gloves may be washed, decontaminated, sterilized, and reused. Utility gloves are used for cleanup and decontamination procedures.

94. (C) Health care workers are at greatest risk for exposure to infection by parenteral transmission of blood-borne pathogens. Parenteral indicates that the pathogen has passed through the skin. Examples include: accidental needlesticks, cuts, and piercing the skin with an instrument.

95. (D) Spiral-shaped bacteria are called spirochetes.

96. (B) A protective barrier plastic wrap is used to cover the head of an x-ray machine.

97. (B) The ultrasonic unit may not remove all forms of bioburden. It is necessary to inspect instruments prior to packaging for sterilization.

98. (A) Glutaraldehyde is EPA registered as a sterilant/disinfectant. If utilized for immersion of instruments that cannot be sterilized by heat, follow manufacturer's instructions for preparation and immerse instruments for 10 hr.

99. (C) *Bacillus subtilis* is the test organism recommended for monitoring dry heat and ethylene oxide sterilizers.

100. (D) The ADA seal of approval is not required on disinfectant labels.

Practice Test Questions 4: Orthodontics

DIRECTIONS (Questions 1–44): Each of the questions or incomplete statements in this section is followed by four suggested answers or completions. Select the **ONE** lettered answer or completion that is **BEST** in each case.

---

1. Orthodontics is the dental specialty that deals with
   A. the diseases and abnormal conditions of the hard and soft tissues of the oral cavity
   B. the treatment of pulpal and periapical diseases of the teeth
   C. the growth and development of the jaws and face
   D. the prevention and education of dental health problems on a community level

2. The condition in which the mandible is located ahead of the maxilla is called
   A. prognathism
   B. micrognathism
   C. retrusion
   D. centric relation

3. The best way to motivate adolescents toward good oral hygiene habits is by
   A. establishing feelings of security
   B. relating it to social acceptance and appearance
   C. explaining monetary considerations
   D. providing a detailed explanation on dental plaque

4. Removal of bands may be accomplished with
   A. a band seater
   B. an explorer
   C. bird-beak pliers
   D. anterior band slitting pliers

5. A headgear appliance is worn
   A. during active play and while sleeping
   B. as the orthodontist prescribes
   C. a minimum of 8 hr. per day, 5 days per week
   D. 24 hr. per day except while eating

6. A positioner is worn
   A. in place of a fixed appliance
   B. for gross tooth movement
   C. to separate the teeth before banding
   D. after the removal of fixed appliances

7. In placing TP springs, an important consideration is
   A. to place them from the lingual surface
   B. to place them from the buccal surface
   C. the placement should be above the contact area
   D. to place them below the contour of the tooth and above the interdental papilla

8. The instrument of choice in ligating an archwire is a
   A. How plier
   B. separating plier
   C. ligature-typing plier
   D. utility plier

9. Direct bracket bonding is advantageous because the procedure
   A. does not add to arch length
   B. permits movement of teeth that will not accept bands
   C. is much more esthetic than traditional cemented brackets
   D. allows the dentist less clinical chair time

10. The attachment either welded or soldered to the bands that secure the archwire is the
   A. bracket
   B. separator

    C. retainer

    D. coil spring

11. Brass separators are removed by

    A. brass separating pliers

    B. cutting opposite the pigtail with ligature cutters

    C. surgical scissors

    D. a sickle scaler

12. What instrument is used to place elastic separators?

    A. Mosquito hemostat

    B. Sickle-type scaler

    C. Elastic separating pliers

    D. Ligature pliers

13. The patient should be instructed to clean his or her retainer

    A. with an electric toothbrush

    B. using hot water

    C. with an immersion agent

    D. after each meal

14. Cephalometry is

    A. taking measurements of the skull

    B. compression of the skull

    C. the study of the soft tissues of the head

    D. a technique of maintaining orthodontic movement

15. Cephalometric tracings are made over

    A. silk screens

    B. extraoral radiographs

    C. articulating paper

    D. special acetate paper

16. The cephalometric headplate taken most often is the

    A. frontal headplate

    B. posteroanterior

    C. lateral skull headplate

    D. cephalostat

17. An open bite refers to a condition wherein
   A. there are no posterior teeth
   B. there are spaces between teeth in the same arch
   C. the anterior teeth do not contact
   D. the teeth contact only during mastication

18. Overjet is the
   A. horizontal distance between maxillary and mandibular teeth
   B. coronal length of maxillary anterior teeth
   C. vertical overlap of maxillary and mandibular anterior teeth
   D. labioversion of the mandibular teeth

19. A type of measuring device commonly used to take intraoral measurements is a (an)
   A. protractor
   B. flexible millimeter ruler
   C. Boone gauge
   D. inch ruler

20. When seating and sizing bands using a band pusher type of instrument, it is necessary to maintain control by
   A. using extraoral finger rests
   B. holding the instrument with both hands
   C. establishing a stable fulcrum before applying pressure
   D. using the patient's chin as support

21. Class III malocclusion is
   A. abnormal crowding of teeth with a normal jaw relationship
   B. a protruded position of the mandible in relation to the maxilla
   C. retruded position of the mandible in relation to maxilla
   D. based on the relationship between maxillary and mandibular second molars

22. Vertical overbite refers to the
   A. horizontal distance between the posterior teeth
   B. coronal length of maxillary anterior teeth
   C. vertical overlap of the incisal edges of maxillary and mandibular anterior teeth
   D. labioversion of mandibular teeth

23. Class II malocclusion is
   A. based on the relationship between maxillary and mandibular first bicuspid
   B. a protruded position of the mandible in relation to the maxilla
   C. also known as neutroclusion
   D. retruded position of the mandible in relation to the maxilla

24. The head-stabilizing device used in cephalometrics is called a (an)
   A. cephalostat
   B. angle board
   C. cassette
   D. articulator

25. During cementation of bands, the cement is placed
   A. on the brackets
   B. on the tooth
   C. on the outer surface of the band
   D. on all surfaces within the band

26. The attachment of anterior plastic brackets directly to teeth can be accomplished by
   A. zinc phosphate cementation
   B. soldering
   C. acid etch bonding
   D. spot welding

27. Cervical anchorage (headgear) is an
   A. appliance that exerts distal forces on maxillary teeth
   B. intraoral appliance that constricts the mandible
   C. intraoral appliance that moves teeth anteriorly
   D. appliance that enlarges the palate

28. After active orthodontic treatment is finished, what appliance is used to stabilize the teeth?
   A. Thin rubber bands
   B. A retainer
   C. A night guard
   D. Molar bands

29. When determining the length of a preformed archwire, you measure the distance from
   A. central to central
   B. first premolar to first premolar
   C. first molar to first molar
   D. tuberosity to tuberosity

30. In the removal of an archwire
   A. ligature ties, then the archwire, are removed one side at a time from the buccal tube
   B. the separators and ligature ties are removed first
   C. the archwire is removed, then the bands are removed
   D. the anterior portion of the archwire is removed before the posterior archwire is removed

31. The most common type of removable retainer is a
   A. headgear appliance
   B. Hawley retainer
   C. positioner
   D. space maintainer

32. What is used to tie the archwire onto orthodontic brackets?
   A. Separating wire
   B. Buccal tubes
   C. Ligature wire
   D. Finger springs

33. When removing separators, care must be taken to
   A. prevent the space from closing too quickly
   B. avoid injuring the interdental papillae
   C. avoid creating too much interdental space
   D. avoid stripping the gingival sulcus

34. A useful instrument for removing elastic separators is
   A. a gold knife
   B. a sharp explorer
   C. crown and collar scissors
   D. a sickle scaler

35. A TP spring is a type of
   A. separator
   B. matrix holder
   C. removable appliance
   D. mouth prop

36. An elastic separator is placed by
   A. snapping through the contacts
   B. gently threading through the contacts with floss threaders
   C. first removing the archwire
   D. stretching and pushing through the contacts

37. When placing an archwire, one should
   A. position the wire into brackets, then guide the wire carefully into the buccal tubes
   B. use a three-pronged plier
   C. insert the wire into one side of the buccal tubes, then guide it into the brackets
   D. use the How pliers

38. The importance of the ligature wire is that it
   A. provides tension for moving teeth
   B. holds the archwire in place
   C. holds brackets on bands
   D. holds the headgear in place

39. When ligating with a tie wire, the tie wire should be
   A. straight
   B. bent at a 45° angle
   C. bent at a 90° angle
   D. applied with a separating plier

40. Select the instrument used to check for loose bands.
   A. Band remover
   B. Bird-beak pliers
   C. How pliers
   D. Pin and ligature pliers

41. After cutting brass wire separators, the pigtails are cut to
  A. 3–5 mm
  B. 1–2 mm
  C. 2–3 mm
  D. the length of the archwire

42. What instrument is used to cut ligature ties in the removal of an archwire?
  A. Pin and ligature cutters
  B. Mosquito forceps
  C. Explorer
  D. Band removing pliers

43. When placing headgear
  A. always ligate to molar tubes
  B. insert one side of facebow first, then the other
  C. pull facebow upward till it snaps into place
  D. make sure inner bow is resting on top of lower lip

44. The type of appliance that has cemented bands and lingual or labial archwires is referred to as
  A. a fixed appliance
  B. a removable appliance
  C. a Hawley appliance
  D. a Crozat appliance

DIRECTIONS (Questions 45–59): For each of the items in this section, **ONE** or **MORE** of the numbered options is correct. Choose answer
  A. if only 1, 2, and 3 are correct
  B. if only 1 and 3 are correct
  C. if only 2 and 4 are correct
  D. if only 4 is correct
  E. if all are correct

---

45. If an orthodontic elastic separator has been swallowed or has disappeared, the assistant should
  1. look for the elastic separator in the oral cavity
  2. call a physician
  3. inform the dentist if it is not located in the oral cavity
  4. do nothing—losing elastic is not important

46. To check for loose bands
1. use band remover pliers to see if cementation is complete
2. look at the bands to see if one is higher or lower than the rest
3. ask the patient if he or she has any loose bands
4. use the How pliers in an occlusal and gingival direction to see if the band moves

47. Which of the following is (are) used to determine if an alginate impression tray is the correct size for the maxillary arch?
1. Tray must extend slightly mesial to the last molar
2. Tray extends to cover the maxillary tuberosity
3. Tray must extend slightly to the floor of the mouth
4. Tray should fit well up into the periphery

48. When inspecting and evaluating an alginate impression, the assistant must check for which of the following?
1. Surface detail
2. Proper extension over retromolar area and peripheral roll
3. Deficiencies in the peripheral impression
4. Final impression has a granular surface

49. The brass separating wire should **NOT** interfere with
1. occlusion
2. gingival tissue
3. chewing
4. speech

50. Which of the following is (are) the correct procedure(s) for mixing zinc phosphate cement for band seating?
1. Spatulate over a large area of slab
2. Mix to putty consistency
3. Use a cool slab
4. Incorporate large increments of powder into the mix

51. The information needed for the diagnosis and treatment planning of an orthodontic case includes
1. complete medical history
2. radiographs and tracings
3. study models
4. photographs

52. An important function of the dental assistant in an orthodontic practice is
1. to keep instruments well sharpened
2. to administer fluoride treatments
3. to chart existing restorations
4. to motivate and reinforce oral hygiene home care

53. A finished Hawley retainer may have
1. an acrylic palate
2. a labial wire
3. arrow clasps
4. a split palate

54. Before cementation
1. brackets are waxed
2. bands are arranged in cementation order
3. teeth are isolated and dried
4. teeth are coronal polished

55. Orthodontic bands with metallic bracket attachments are designed to be
1. placed on occlusal surfaces of the teeth
2. cemented on teeth to hold the cervical neck collar
3. held in place by elastic and finger springs
4. cemented on teeth as a means of anchoring archwires

56. In reference to an orthodontic study cast model
1. trimmed models must be polished and labeled
2. a model trimmer is used to establish right angles
3. white orthodontic plaster is used
4. wax bite is used to occlude models while trimming the heel

57. If an archwire does not go in
1. check for a crushed bracket
2. the molar band tube is blocked
3. check width and diameter of archwire
4. check the tongue

58. In the placement and removal of elastic ligatures, which of the following instruments may be used?
  1. Locking hemostat
  2. Pigtail explorer
  3. Scaler
  4. Ligature-tying pliers

59. After removal of the orthodontic bands, all excess cement should be removed because
  1. gingival irritation may occur
  2. teeth will not occlude properly
  3. teeth may appear discolored
  4. cement is irritating to the interproximal surfaces of teeth

---

DIRECTIONS (Questions 60–72): Refer to Figures 4–1 through 4–8 to answer the following questions.

---

60. Identify the instrument shown in Figure 4–1.
  A. Rubber dam clamp forceps
  B. Ligature-tying pliers
  C. Separating pliers
  D. Mosquito hemostat

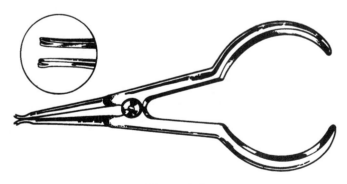

Figure 4–1

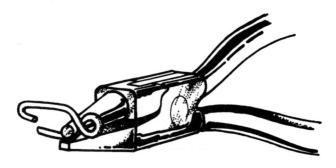

Figure 4–2

61. Identify the orthodontic instrument shown in Figure 4–2.
   A. Elastic separator
   B. Brass wire separator
   C. Coil spring
   D. TP spring

62. The orthodontic pliers shown in Figure 4–3 are designed primarily for
   A. removal of orthodontic bands
   B. attachment of ortho brackets
   C. removal of headgear
   D. cementation of ortho bands

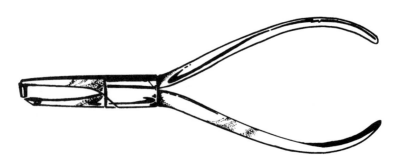

Figure 4–3

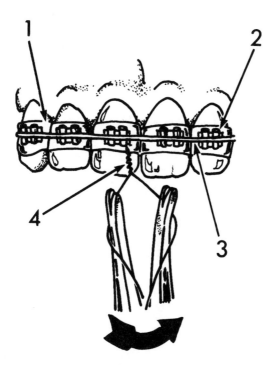

Figure 4–4

63. Locate the orthodontic bracket in Figure 4–4.
   A. 1
   B. 2
   C. 3
   D. Not shown

64. Locate the orthodontic archwire in Figure 4–4.
   A. 1
   B. 2
   C. 3
   D. 4

65. Locate the orthodontic tie wire in Figure 4–4.
   A. 1
   B. 2
   C. 3
   D. 4

66. Locate the headgear tube in Figure 4–4.
- **A.** 1
- **B.** 2
- **C.** 3
- **D.** Not shown

67. Locate the orthodontic band in Figure 4–4.
- **A.** 1
- **B.** 2
- **C.** 3
- **D.** Not shown

68. Figure 4–5 indicates placement of a (an)
- **A.** positioner
- **B.** elastic separator
- **C.** elastic rubber band
- **D.** separating wire

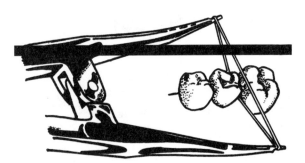

Figure 4–5

69. In reference to Figure 4–6, all of the following are true **EXCEPT**
- **A.** the high-pull headgear does not require a facebow
- **B.** headgear appliances must not be worn during contact sports
- **C.** the cervical neck band design is attached to the outer facebow by hooks
- **D.** the number of hours the headgear is to be worn is determined by the doctor

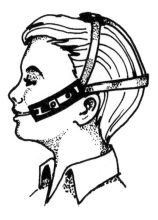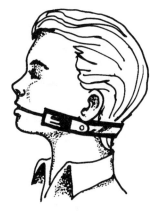

Figure 4–6

70. The primary function of the cervical facebow shown in Figure 4–7 is to
   A. stabilize an extraoral radiograph
   B. serve as an anchor for the mandibular archwire
   C. apply direct force to the maxillary molars and restrain maxillary anterior growth
   D. apply direct force to the lower lip and mandibular arch

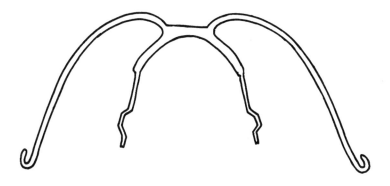

Figure 4–7

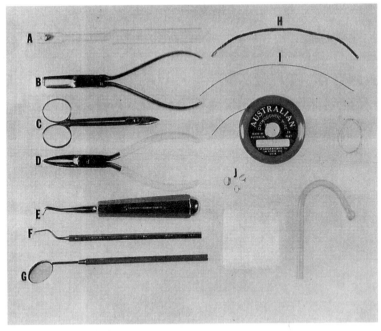

Figure 4–8

71. Identify the orthodontic bands, band pusher, and ligature wire in Figure 4–8.
  A. I, D, and A
  B. H, I, and F
  C. B, H, and D
  D. J, E, and H

72. Identify the band removing pliers, band seater, and scaler in Figure 4–8.
  A. A, D, and I
  B. B, A, and F
  C. D, H, and C
  D. E, B, and J

DIRECTIONS (Questions 73–77): Match the oral physiotherapy devices in Column A with their functions in Column B.

COLUMN A   **COLUMN B**

73. floss holder _____   **A.** effective for large interproximal
74. disclosing agent _____   areas and fixed bridges
75. perio aid _____   **B.** cleanses under gingival margins
76. balsawood cleaner _____   and root furcations
77. interdental brush _____   **C.** recommended for teeth with
                           gingival recession
                       D. effective in identifying plaque
                       E. assists patients with limited dexterity

DIRECTIONS (Questions 78–85): Each of the questions or incomplete statements in this section is followed by four suggested answers or completions. Select the **ONE** lettered answer or completion that is **BEST** in each case.

78. On which surface(s) is the archwire located?
   A. Incisal surfaces only
   B. Labial surfaces only
   C. Lingual surfaces only
   D. Labial or lingual surface

79. One of the most important tasks of the assistant when attempting to support an anxious patient is to be
   A. efficient
   B. calm and cool
   C. centered
   D. strong

80. A water irrigator is used
   A. to remove plaque
   B. as a substitute for a toothbrush
   C. to remove loose food debris
   D. as a substitute for dental floss

81. To be of maximum benefit to the teeth, the optimum fluoride concentration is
   A. 10%
   B. 1 ppm
   C. 100 ppm
   D. 2 ppm

82. Which of the following are considered detergent foods?
   A. Bananas
   B. Raisins
   C. Cheese
   D. Apples

83. Using the heel or toe of the brush is helpful for cleaning which tooth surfaces?
   A. Buccal surfaces of molars
   B. Lingual surfaces of molars
   C. Lingual surfaces of anterior teeth
   D. Facial surfaces of anterior teeth

84. According to the manufacturer, regular preventive maintenance for the model trimmer includes all of the following **EXCEPT**
   A. replace rag wheels
   B. check water hoses for leaks
   C. periodic replacement of abrasive grinding wheels
   D. maintain model trimmer work platform plaster free

85. Gypsum materials used for orthodontic procedures are best stored in a
   A. locked storage bin
   B. airtight dry container
   C. lead-lined open container
   D. biohazard plastic container

Practice Test Questions 4: Orthodontics

Answers and Discussion

1. **(C)** Orthodontics is the dental specialty that deals with the growth and development of the jaws and face. Treatment includes correction of occlusion and facial contour.

2. **(A)** Prognathism is the condition in which the mandible is located ahead of the maxilla. The correction of this bony defect is a combination of surgery and orthodontic treatment. The mandible is cut bilaterally and moved posteriorly to a position of desired occlusion. The mandible is then stabilized for approximately 6 weeks.

3. **(B)** The best way to motivate adolescents toward good oral hygiene habits is by emphasizing the relationship between good daily oral hygiene and both social acceptance and appearance.

4. **(D)** Removal of bands may be accomplished with anterior band slitting pliers, posterior band removing pliers, or both.

5. **(B)** A headgear appliance is to be worn as the orthodontist prescribes. Most headgear appliances are worn 24 hr. per day except while eating. The headgear appliance is accompanied by a wired facebow. The headgear appliance may encircle the neck or the head or both. The patient must be cautioned not to engage in contact sports while using orthodontic headgear.

6. (D) A positioner is worn after orthodontic treatment has been completed. The primary function of the orthodontic positioner is to allow the alveolar bone to become stronger around the teeth before the patient wears an orthodontic retainer. The patient is instructed to wear the appliance for long periods of time and to exercise the jaws by chewing up and down vigorously.

7. (A) Steel spring separators, such as TP springs, should be inserted from the lingual surface and below the contact point of the tooth.

8. (C) The instrument of choice in ligating an archwire is the ligature-tying plier. The hemostat occasionally is used to tighten or twist the archwire.

9. (D) Direct bracket bonding is advantageous because the procedure allows the dentist less clinical chair time.

10. (A) Brackets are either welded or soldered to the orthodontic bands. Anterior band brackets differ from molar brackets (buccal tubes) on orthodontic bands.

11. (B) Brass separators are removed by cutting with a ligature cutter or wire cutter. Avoid trauma to soft gingival tissues when removing brass separators.

12. (C) Elastic separating pliers are used to place elastic separators.

13. (D) The patient should be instructed to clean the retainer after every meal. Toothpaste and cold water or a mild soap and cold water may be used to brush off soft deposits.

14. (A) Cephalometry is the part of orthodontic diagnosis that studies the measurement of the skull to determine skeletal patterns. The measurements are taken from tracings of extraoral radiographs (lateral plates and posteroanterior plates).

15. (B) Cephalometric tracings are made over extraoral radiographs on special acetate paper or orthodontic tracing paper. Landmarks of the skull are transferred onto the orthodontic tracing paper with a white tracing pencil.

16. (C) The cephalometric headplate taken most often is the lateral skull headplate.

17. (C) An open bite refers to an orthodontic problem wherein the anterior teeth do not contact each other. The etiology may be a habit, such as thumbsucking or tongue thrusting. The treatment may include discontinuance of the habit and orthodontic intervention.

18. (A) Overjet, also known as horizontal overbite, is the horizontal distance between the incisal edges of the maxillary and mandibular anterior teeth when they are in occlusion.

19. (B) A type of measuring device commonly used to take intraoral measurements is the flexible millimeter ruler. The protractor is used to make cephalometric tracings. The Boone gauge is used to measure the height of orthodontic bands.

20. (C) When seating and sizing bands using a band pusher type of instrument, it is necessary to maintain control by establishing a stable fulcrum before applying pressure. A stable fulcrum prevents accidental slippage and laceration of the soft tissues. An intraoral fulcrum close to the working site should always be maintained.

21. (B) Class III malocclusion, or mesioclusion, indicates that the mesiobuccal cusp of the maxillary first molar occludes in the interdental space between the distal cusp of the mandibular first permanent molar and the mesial cusp of the mandibular second permanent molar, giving the appearance of a protruded mandible in relation to the maxilla.

22. (C) Vertical overbite refers to the vertical overlap of the incisal edges of the maxillary and mandibular anterior teeth when the teeth are in occlusion.

23. (D) Class II malocclusion is also known as distoclusion. Class II malocclusion indicates that the mesial-buccal cusp of the maxillary first molar is mesial to the buccal groove of the mandibular first molar, giving the appearance of a retruded mandible in relation to the maxilla.

24. **(A)** The head-stabilizing device used for cephalometric radiography is called a cephalostat or cephalometer.

25. **(D)** During cementation of orthodontic bands, the cement is mixed to a creamy consistency and placed on all surfaces within the band. At least two bands are filled with cement simultaneously during the cementation procedure.

26. **(C)** Acid etch bonding is currently used to attach clear plastic brackets directly to anterior teeth. This technique is more esthetically pleasing to many patients than the metal bands and brackets.

27. **(A)** Cervical anchorage is an appliance that attaches intraorally to the maxillary molars and protrudes extraorally to attach to an elastic band that fits around the patient's neck. This appliance provides distal forces to move the molars.

28. **(B)** After orthodontic treatment is finished, a retainer is used to stabilize the teeth in the correct position.

29. **(C)** When determining the length of a preformed archwire, you measure the distance from first molar to first molar.

30. **(A)** In the removal of an archwire, the ligatures, then the archwire, are removed one side at a time from the buccal tube.

31. **(B)** The Hawley retainer is the most common type of orthodontic removable appliance. The Hawley retainer is made of clear acrylic and contouring wire and is worn after removal of orthodontic bands to maintain teeth in their new position. The Hawley retainer is also used for minor orthodontic corrections of the teeth.

32. **(C)** Ligature wire is used to tie the archwire into brackets. Rubber bands can also be used to hold the archwire in the brackets and tubes.

33. **(B)** When removing separators, care must be taken to avoid injuring the interdental papillae.

34. **(D)** A useful instrument for removing elastic separators is the sickle scaler. The sickle scaler is used to gently lift the elastic sep-

arator away from the contact area of the teeth. The elastic separator should be removed in an occlusal direction. A stable fulcrum point is necessary to prevent injury to the soft tissues. The number of elastic separators removed must correspond to the number of separators originally placed.

35. (A) A TP spring is a type of orthodontic separator. Orthodontic separators are placed between the teeth before orthodontic banding procedures to allow for adequate separation of the teeth when the bands are ready to be cemented. Separators may be made of elastic or wire.

36. (D) An elastic separator is placed with the elastic separating pliers by stretching and pushing through the contacts of the teeth in a buccolingual motion. Correct placement should be checked with a mouth mirror and explorer.

37. (C) When placing an archwire, one should insert the archwire into one side of the buccal tubes, then guide it into the brackets. The same procedure is repeated on the other side.

38. (B) The ligature tie wire is a fine-gauge wire used to tie the main preformed archwire onto the brackets of the cemented orthodontic bands. Ligature wire holds the archwire securely in place.

39. (B) Ligature tie wires are applied with ligature tying pliers. A tie wire loop is bent at a 45° angle and carefully inserted over and around the fixed bracket of the orthodontic band. The wire is guided behind the bracket and over the archwire, ligated to 4 mm, then cut with ligature cutters to a 2-mm pigtail. The ends are tucked under to avoid irritation to the soft tissues.

40. (C) The How pliers are used to check for loose orthodontic bands.

41. (C) After cutting brass wire separators, the pigtails are cut to approximately 2–3 mm long. The free end of the pigtail is then tucked in a gingival direction with a condenser type of instrument.

42. (A) Pin and ligature cutters (pliers) are used to cut ligature ties for the removal of an archwire. The cut should be made as close to the pigtail as possible. After snipping the wire, use a hemostat to pull it free. Instruct the patient to keep eyes closed during the procedure to avoid accidental injury to the eye. Protective eyewear should be worn by the assistant.

43. **(B)** When placing headgear, insert one side of the inner facebow first, then the other side. Once the inner facebow is in place, apply straps over the hooks for placement of the outer bow of the headgear appliance.

44. **(A)** A fixed appliance has cemented bands and a lingual or labial archwire. The Hawley and Crozat appliances are designed to be removable.

45. **(B)** If an orthodontic elastic separator has been swallowed or has disappeared, the assistant should look for the elastic separator by examining the oral cavity and inform the dentist of the missing separator.

46. **(D)** To check for loose bands, examine the mouth carefully to see if bands are properly aligned and use the How plier in an occlusal and gingival direction to see if the orthodontic band moves.

47. **(C)** If an alginate impression tray is the correct size for the maxillary arch, the tray should extend to cover the maxillary tuberosity and fit well up into the periphery to obtain the proper study cast model.

48. **(A)** When inspecting and evaluating an alginate impression, the assistant must check for surface detail, proper extension over retromolar area and periphery borders, and any type of surface deficiencies or impression discrepancies.

49. **(E)** Brass separators should be placed carefully in the mouth so as not to interfere with occlusion, gingival tissues, chewing, or speech.

50. **(B)** When mixing zinc phosphate cement for band seating, use a cool glass slab approximately 70° F and spatulate cement over a large area of the slab to dissipate heat. Mix enough cement to a creamy consistency for multiple band seating.

51. (E) To diagnose and plan treatment for an orthodontic case, it is necessary to have a complete medical history, extraoral radiographs, cephalometric tracings, study models, and photographs showing facial profiles.

52. (D) An important function of the dental assistant in an orthodontic practice is to motivate and reinforce home oral hygiene care and plaque control. Patient education in proper nutrition and maintenance and care of orthodontic appliances is also a responsibility of the orthodontic dental assistant.

53. (A) A finished Hawley retainer may have an acrylic palate, labial archwire, and arrow clasps. The Crozat appliance (or jackscrew) has a split palate design to widen a narrow palate.

54. (E) Before cementation of bands, brackets must be waxed, teeth must be thoroughly polished and dried, and the orthodontic bands must be arranged in the order of cementation.

55. (D) Orthodontic bands with metallic bracket attachments are designed to be cemented on the teeth and serve as a support for anchoring and stabilizing the orthodontic archwires.

56. (E) In reference to an orthodontic study cast model, the impressions should be poured in white orthodontic plaster of Paris. Models are trimmed on a model trimmer and are occluded together while trimming the heels of the maxillary and mandibular cast. A wax bite is used to prevent accidental fracture of the teeth during this trimming procedure. Orthodontic study models must be polished and labeled properly, including the patient's full name and age and the date.

57. (A) If an archwire does not go in properly, check for a crushed bracket, possible blocked molar tube, and inadequate length of archwire.

58. (B) Elastic ligatures are placed over the bracket wings once the archwire has been secured. Hemostats may be used for application. Removal of the elastic ligatures is done with a sickle scaler. Ligature-tying pliers are used for anchoring ligature tie wires only.

59. (E) Teeth should be thoroughly scaled and polished after removal of cemented orthodontic bands. Excess residual cement will cause gingival irritation and be visibly unaesthetic, causing possible discoloration of the teeth. Occlusion and contacts are also affected by residual cement deposits. Appropriate oral hygiene instructions should be given to the patient immediately after orthodontic treatment.

60. (B)

61. (D)

62. (A)

63. (B)

64. (C)

65. (D)

66. (D)

67. (A)

68. (B)

69. (A)

70. (C)

71. (D)

72. (B)

73. (E)

74. (D)

75. (B)

76. (C)

77. (A)

78. (D) The archwire can be located on either the labial or lingual surface. When activated, an archwire applies force to slowly move teeth.

79. (C) The anxious patient needs to test reality. The assistant must give the patient his or her complete attention and not become distracted by other events occurring in the office.

80. (C) Water irrigators are used to remove loose debris.

81. (B) The optimum amount of fluoride in drinking water is 1 ppm. The process of adding fluoride to the drinking water is called fluoridation.

82. (D) Apples are considered to be detergent foods and assist in removing sticky food debris. Detergent foods help to stimulate the gingival tissues. Orthodontic patients should avoid hard, crunchy foods which may injure delicate appliances.

83. (C) The heel and toe of a soft bristle toothbrush are most effective in cleaning lingual surfaces of anterior teeth, since these areas are narrow and curved.

84. (A) Rag wheels are not part of a model trimmer. The rag wheels are used with a dental lathe for polishing.

85. (B) Gypsum products are best stored in a cool area housed in an airtight dry container. When working around gypsum products personal protective equipment (ppe) is recommended to prevent inhalation of gypsum powder and irritation to the eyes. A warning label should be affixed to the secondary container housing the gypsum products in accordance with the OSHA Hazard Communication Standard.

Practice Test Questions 5: Oral and Maxillofacial Surgery

DIRECTIONS (Questions 1–10): Each of the numbered items or incomplete statements in this section is followed by four suggested answers or completions. Select the **ONE** lettered answer or completion that is **BEST** in each case.

---

1. An impaction is
   A. a succedaneous tooth
   B. a tooth that will not erupt fully
   C. any tooth that is ankylosed
   D. a supernumerary tooth

2. The basic components of a surgical elevator are
   A. handle, shank, and tip
   B. handle, hinge, and beak
   C. handle, shank, and beak
   D. handle, shank, and point

3. Rongeurs forceps are designed for
   A. gross bone removal
   B. splitting teeth in bone
   C. cutting and contouring bone
   D. removing root tips

4. An instrument that holds a tissue flap away from the operating field is called a
   A. pick
   B. retractor
   C. elevator
   D. hemostat

5. A biopsy is
   A. any lesion in the oral cavity
   B. the surgical removal of an abscessed tooth
   C. the removal of tissue for diagnostic purposes
   D. the radical removal of a cancerous lesion

6. Surgical burs are specifically designed with
   A. prepackaged sterile pouches
   B. extra long shanks
   C. long cutting blades
   D. pretreated metal alloys

7. The basic components of an extraction forcep are
   A. handle, shank, and tip
   B. handle, hinge, and beak
   C. handle, shank, and beak
   D. handle, shank, and point

8. General anesthetics are administered
   A. for nerve blocks
   B. routinely in most dental offices
   C. to render the patient unconscious
   D. without any risks

9. Before assisting in surgery in the hospital operating room the assistant should perform a thorough surgical scrub for approximately
   A. 1 min.
   B. 3 min.
   C. 5 min.
   D. 10 min.

10. Instrument transfer of surgical forceps is done using a
    A. two-handed palm grasp
    B. one-handed modified pen grasp

    C. two-handed pen grasp
    D. stable fulcrum

DIRECTIONS (Question 11–15): Match each item in Column A with the appropriate explanation in Column B.

COLUMN A

11. local anesthesia   _____
12. general anesthesia _____
13. nitrous oxide   _____
14. intravenous
    sedation   _____
15. narcotic analgesic _____

COLUMN B

A. weakest of the inhalation anesthetic agents
B. primarily intravenous barbiturates as a group
C. vasoconstrictors that allow profound analgesia, remove pain but not pressure sensation
D. induces loss of sensation and consciousness
E. leaves patient conscious but extremely drowsy, reduces state of awareness and anxiety

---

DIRECTIONS (Questions 16–39): Each of the questions or incomplete statements in this section is followed by four suggested answers or completions. Select the **ONE** lettered answer or completion that is **BEST** in each case.

---

16. Monitoring a patient during general anesthesia or intravenous sedation is the primary responsibility of the
    A. surgeon
    B. Certified Dental Assistant
    C. surgical team
    D. monitoring surgical assistant

17. The three body systems that are monitored on a patient during general anesthesia or intravenous sedation are the
    A. cardiovascular, lymphatic, and peripheral systems
    B. cardiovascular, central venous, and muscular systems
    C. cardiovascular, central nervous, and respiratory systems
    D. digestive, respiratory, and lymphatic systems

18. The pulse is monitored by palpating the
   A. radial or carotid veins
   B. radial or temporal arteries
   C. radial or carotid arteries
   D. carotid or temporal veins

19. When palpating the pulse, you should be aware of the
   A. location, placement, and strength of the pulse
   B. rate, rhythm, and strength of the pulse
   C. respiration rate per minute
   D. patient's body temperature

20. The characteristics of a laryngospasm are
   A. snoring, gurgling, and high-pitched crowing
   B. snoring, gasping, and high-pitched crowing
   C. gasping, sneezing, and high-pitched crowing
   D. gurgling, wheezing, and high-pitched crowing

21. The electrocardiogram is a graphic tracing of the electrical activity of the
   A. brain
   B. pulse
   C. central nervous system
   D. heart

22. After surgery, the patient is instructed not to drink liquids using a straw because it may cause
   A. premature healing
   B. a dry socket
   C. bleeding to occur
   D. an initial infection

23. Intravenous barbiturates are classified as
   A. analgesics
   B. anesthetics
   C. sedative-hypnotics
   D. unconscious producing hypnotics

24. The greatest potential danger of a narcotic analgesic is depression of the
   A. central nervous system
   B. respiratory system
   C. cardiovascular system
   D. peripheral system

25. Common complications that may occur during the postoperative recovery period are
   A. respiratory obstruction, bodily injury, and hemorrhage
   B. abdominal pain, vomiting, and giddiness
   C. gastroenteritis and elevated blood pressure
   D. vomiting and postoperative pain

26. The most common complication associated with implants is the lack of
   A. good oral hygiene
   B. osseointegration
   C. gingival support
   D. patient compliance

27. Which of the following metals used for implants possesses favorable biomechanical and biocompatible properties?
   A. Titanium
   B. Surgical silver
   C. Stainless steel
   D. Carbonium

28. Dental implants are classified in which of the following three categories?
   A. Endosteal, periosteal, and transosteal implants
   B. Subperiosteal, transosteal, and subendosteal implants
   C. Endosteal, subperiosteal, and transosteal implants
   D. Subperiosteal, endosteal, and subtransosteal implants

29. The most common general anesthetic agents used in oral and maxillofacial surgery are
   A. Anectine and Brevital
   B. Brevital and Diprivan
   C. Valium and Brevital
   D. atropine sulfate and Brevital

30. A narcotic antagonist drug is
   A. Vistaril
   B. flumazenil
   C. atropine
   D. naxolone

31. The treatment of fractures is
   A. the placement of a drain
   B. immediate mobilization
   C. immobilization
   D. bony transplants

32. The Caldwell-Luc procedure is performed to remove a
   A. full bony impacted tooth
   B. partial bony impacted tooth
   C. displaced mesiodens
   D. displaced tooth in the maxillary sinus

33. A hand instrument used for gross bone removal and to split teeth is called a
   A. periosteal elevator
   B. surgical chisel
   C. surgical bur
   D. rongeurs

34. An instrument used to effectively remove debris and diseased tissue from a tooth socket is a
   A. surgical curette
   B. scalpel
   C. elevator
   D. curved hemostat

35. An elevator instrument is designed to luxate and remove
   A. impacted wisdom teeth
   B. deciduous teeth
   C. root tip fragments only
   D. roots, teeth, and root tip fragments

36. A particular elevator used to loosen the gingival tissue surrounding the tooth before an extraction is the
   A. angular elevator
   B. periosteal elevator
   C. cross-bar elevator
   D. east-west elevator

37. A drain is placed in a surgical site to
   A. hold bone fractures together
   B. treat gingival grafts
   C. treat dry sockets
   D. create a pathway for fluid to leave the body

38. Before dismissing a patient immediately after surgery, the dental assistant must check the patient for all of the following **EXCEPT**
   A. swelling
   B. excessive bleeding
   C. dizziness
   D. postoperative instructions have been read and reviewed

39. Nitrous oxide is used primarily in oral surgery as
   A. a local anesthetic
   B. an inhalation sedation agent
   C. a sedative agent to bring the patient to an unconscious state
   D. an inhalation agent to assist the patient with respiratory problems

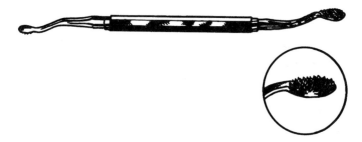

Figure 5–1

DIRECTIONS (Questions 40–53): Refer to Figures 5–1 through 5–14 to answer the following questions.

---

40. Identify the instrument shown in Figure 5–1.
    A. Bone file
    B. Chisel
    C. Tissue retractor
    D. Surgical curette

41. The instrument shown in Figure 5–2 is designed primarily to
    A. stabilize implant abutments
    B. clamp blood vessels and arteries
    C. hold a suture needle
    D. extract deciduous teeth

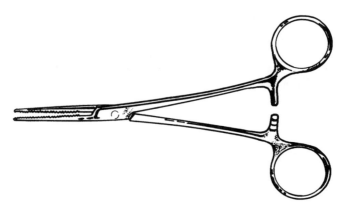

Figure 5–2

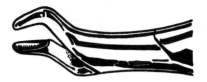

Figure 5–3

42. The surgical tips of the forceps shown in Figure 5–3 are used to extract which teeth?
    A. The mandibular third molars
    B. The maxillary molars
    C. The maxillary anteriors
    D. The mandibular anteriors

43. Identify the instrument shown in Figure 5–4.
    A. Rongeur
    B. Periosteal elevator
    C. Crossbar elevator
    D. Cryer elevator

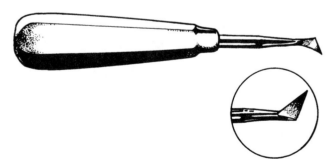

Figure 5–4

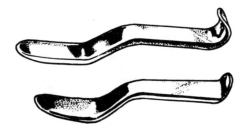

Figure 5–5

44. The instruments shown in Figure 5–5 are designed primarily for
    A. surgical biopsies requiring bone removal
    B. soft tissue retraction
    C. elevation of periodontally involved teeth
    D. taking intraoral photographs

45. Identify the No. 12 surgical blade in Figure 5–6.
    A.
    B.
    C.
    D. The No. 12 surgical blade is not shown

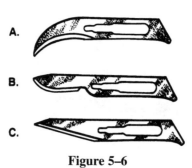

Figure 5–6

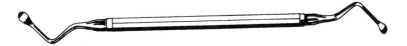

Figure 5–7

46. The instrument shown in Figure 5–7 is designed primarily to
  A. remove a suture
  B. place periodontal dressings
  C. remove necrotic tissues
  D. place postextraction dressings

47. The primary function of the forceps shown in Figure 5–8 is
  A. to remove palatal tori
  B. to cut alveolar bone
  C. to remove maxillary anterior teeth
  D. to remove mandibular anterior teeth

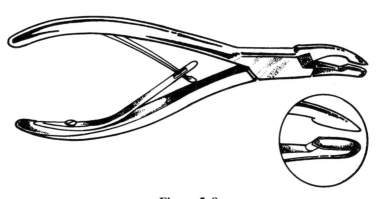

Figure 5–8

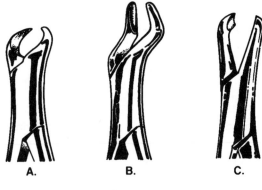

Figure 5–9

48. The No. 23 cowhorn surgical forcep is used to remove mandibular molars. Identify the No. 23 cowhorn surgical forcep in Figure 5–9.
   A.
   B.
   C.
   D. No. 23 forcep is not shown

49. The forcep shown in Figure 5–10 is designed to extract
   A. maxillary anterior teeth
   B. mandibular first primary molars
   C. mandibular primary second molars
   D. mandibular first molars

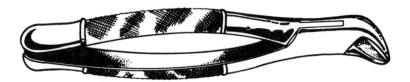

Figure 5–10

A.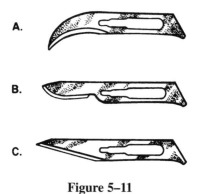

B.

C.

Figure 5–11

50. Identify the No. 15 surgical blade in Figure 5–11.
    A.
    B.
    C.
    D. No. 15 surgical blade is not shown

51. The instrument shown in Figure 5–12 is designed primarily to
    A. loosen the tooth from the bony socket
    B. remove cysts
    C. recontour bone
    D. separate fused roots

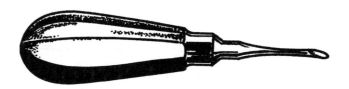

Figure 5–12

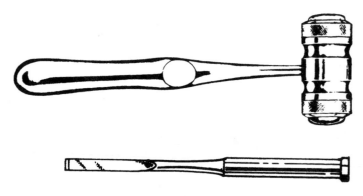

Figure 5–13

52. The surgical mallet and chisel shown in Figure 5–13 are used specifically during surgical procedures for
   A. dental implants
   B. resetting fractured mandibles
   C. bone removal and recontouring
   D. removal of posterior teeth

53. Identify the instrument shown in Figure 5–14.
   A. Surgical curette
   B. Periosteal elevator
   C. Straight elevator
   D. Bone file

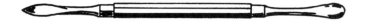

Figure 5–14

DIRECTIONS (Questions 54–57): Match the lettered illustration in Figure 5–15 with the corresponding question.

54. Identify the needle holder, bone file, and syringe.
   A. A, H, and L
   B. C, E, and F
   C. D, G, and K
   D. I, J, and L

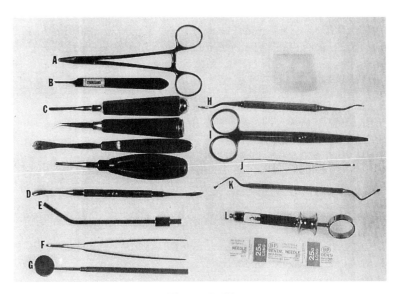

Figure 5–15

55. Identify the surgical curette, straight elevator, and tissue forceps.
   A. B, C, and I
   B. K, C, and F
   C. E, H, and J
   D. G, I, and L

56. Identify the tissue forceps, scissors, and scalpel.
   A. J, L, and B
   B. D, G, and L
   C. E, H, and K
   D. F, K, and L

57. Identify the surgical suction, mouth mirror, and periosteal elevator.
   A. C, E, and G
   B. K, H, and E
   C. E, G, and D
   D. H, G, and D

DIRECTIONS (Questions 58–86): Each of the questions or incomplete statements in this section is followed by four suggested answers or completions. Select the **ONE** lettered answer or completion that is **BEST** in each case.

---

58. Health history questionnaires must be completed
   A. at every dental appointment
   B. before rendering clinical dental care
   C. in ink at the end of the dental treatment
   D. only if a surgical procedure is indicated

59. A patient dental record provides information on all of the following **EXCEPT**
   A. lab biopsy results
   B. EKG monitoring reports
   C. universal precautions
   D. drug allergies

60. When taking a blood pressure reading, the first sound heard is the
   A. diastolic pressure
   B. systolic pressure
   C. carotid pressure
   D. pulse pressure

61. The color of the oxygen cylinder tank is always
   A. green
   B. blue
   C. red
   D. white

62. The lower edge of the sphygmomanometer cuff is positioned
   A. 2″ above the crease of the elbow
   B. 4″ above the crease of the elbow
   C. 1″ above the crease of the elbow
   D. 1″ below the crease of the elbow

63. The average resting pulse rate for an adult is
   A. 40–50 beats per minute
   B. 60–100 beats per minute

    C. 120–140 beats per minute
    D. 150 beats per minute

64. A normal oral temperature reading for a healthy adult is
    A. 98.6° F
    B. 96.8° F
    C. 100° F
    D. 101° F

65. Normal respiratory rate per minute for an adult is
    A. 10–12 breaths per minute
    B. 12–14 breaths per minute
    C. 14–16 breaths per minute
    D. 16–20 breaths per minute

66. The amount of air that cannot be expirated from the lungs is called the
    A. tidal air
    B. residual air
    C. vital capacity
    D. alveolar air

67. Medical emergencies can be prevented by
    A. thoroughly charting all existing oral conditions
    B. presetting instrument trays
    C. keeping the operatory as sterile as possible
    D. being alert to signs and symptoms of impending emergencies

68. Short appointments are given to patients with a history of
    A. allergies
    B. cardiac problems
    C. aphthous ulcers
    D. rampant caries

69. The depressed state of many body functions is called
    A. shock
    B. depression
    C. psychosis
    D. mental retardation

70. When treating for shock, the body position is
  A. head lower than the rest of the body
  B. based on the injury
  C. head and shoulders raised 8–12″
  D. flat, with head turned to the side

71. Syncope refers to
  A. a sudden state of excitement
  B. loss of consciousness
  C. dizziness after an injection
  D. hypertension

72. Inhalation of spirits of ammonia is used to treat
  A. insulin shock
  B. respiratory collapse
  C. circulatory collapse
  D. syncope

73. If a patient faints, the assistant should
  A. seat the patient upright
  B. place the head lower than the rest of the body
  C. hold the patient's head in his or her lap
  D. sharply slap the patient's face

74. Chronic respiratory problems affect the
  A. type of prosthesis a patient can wear
  B. prognosis of root canal therapy
  C. positioning of the patient in the dental chair
  D. type of x-rays taken

75. The proper sequence in an emergency situation is
  A. treat for shock, control severe bleeding, restore breathing
  B. restore breathing, treat for shock, control severe bleeding
  C. restore breathing, control severe bleeding, treat for shock
  D. control severe bleeding, restore breathing, treat for shock

76. If circulatory collapse occurs, the patient should be
  A. given a drink of warm water
  B. left alone
  C. given external cardiac massage
  D. seated upright

77. Proper preparation of a victim for artificial respiration is to
   A. wipe foreign matter from mouth and tilt head backward with chin pointing downward
   B. wipe foreign matter from mouth and tilt head backward with chin pointing upward
   C. tilt head backward with chin pointing upward, put one hand under victim's neck and lift
   D. do not wipe foreign matter from mouth but lift victim's neck to raise chin

78. Anaphylactic shock is
   A. a chronic allergic condition
   B. the result of aspirating a foreign object
   C. a sudden violent allergic reaction
   D. a reaction to mental depression

79. The drug that best counteracts anaphylactic shock is
   A. Novocain
   B. Xylocaine
   C. epinephrine
   D. a barbiturate

80. A patient taking anticoagulation medication could pose a problem related to
   A. the length of the appointment
   B. hemorrhage control
   C. stress and anxiety of the dental situation
   D. muscular coordination and trismus

81. Symptoms of postural hypotension include
   A. profuse sweating
   B. elevated (high) blood pressure
   C. low blood pressure
   D. a sudden state of excitement

82. To reduce the possibility of injury during an epileptic seizure, the operator or assistant should
    A. remove anything nearby that might get in the way, such as furniture or equipment, and not interfere with the patient during the seizure
    B. place padded tongue depressors between the patient's teeth
    C. attempt to hold the patient absolutely still
    D. seat the patient in a straight-backed chair

83. When performing chest compressions, the heel of the hand should be placed
    A. near the xiphoid process
    B. at the center of the chest just below the heart
    C. two or three finger widths above the lower end of the sternum
    D. just above the heart

84. If a permanent central incisor is accidentally avulsed, what is the treatment?
    A. Throw the tooth away—it cannot be saved
    B. Promptly reinsert tooth and see the dentist immediately
    C. Keep the tooth moist in tap water until medical help can be summoned
    D. Reinsert the tooth and keep teeth as clean as possible

85. Insulin shock is due to
    A. too much blood sugar
    B. too much insulin in the blood
    C. too little insulin in the blood
    D. overeating

86. Medical emergency procedures for a patient going into insulin shock include
    A. have the patient ingest sugar cubes or a sweet drink
    B. give an injection of insulin immediately
    C. place a nitroglycerin tablet sublingually
    D. send the patient home, then call his or her physician

DIRECTIONS (Questions 87–94): For each of the items in this section, **ONE** or **MORE** of the numbered options is correct. Choose answer
- **A.** if only 1, 2, and 3 are correct
- **B.** if only 1 and 3 are correct
- **C.** if only 2 and 4 are correct
- **D.** if only 4 is correct
- **E.** if all are correct

87. Placing a nitroglycerin tablet under the tongue is the suggested emergency treatment for a patient suffering from
1. syncope
2. epilepsy
3. anaphylactic shock
4. angina pectoris

88. Lawsuits can be avoided by
1. keeping accurate and complete records
2. understanding the state Dental Practice Act and its limitations
3. knowing your patient's health history and contraindications
4. obtaining appropriate patient consent before treatment

89. Due to lack of oxygen, brain cells begin to die after
1. 30 sec.
2. 1 min.
3. 2–3 min.
4. 4–6 min.

90. Acetone breath, dry mouth, thirst, and weak pulse are possible symptoms of
1. hypertension
2. epilepsy
3. kidney disease
4. diabetic coma

91. Medical emergency treatment for the patient who is hyperventilating includes which of the following?
1. Have the patient take deep, slow breaths
2. Administer oxygen quickly
3. Place a paper bag over the patient's nose and mouth
4. Have the patient lie down in a supine position

92. Symptoms of a stroke (CVA) may include
1. irregular, thready pulse
2. slurred speech
3. cyanosis
4. generalized body rash

93. A basic office emergency armamentarium includes
1. portable oxygen tanks
2. intravenous armamentarium and related drugs
3. sponges and tourniquets
4. sugar packs

94. The patient with a history of liver disease (hepatitis) should be given which drug in limited quantities?
1. Oxygen
2. Dilantin
3. Nitrous oxide
4. Local anesthetics

DIRECTIONS (Questions 95–115): Each of the questions or incomplete statements in this section is followed by four suggested answers or completions. Select the **ONE** lettered answer or completion that is **BEST** in each case.

---

95. Before prescribing any drug
A. an accurate medical history must be taken
B. a Snyder test should be performed
C. a complete blood count should be performed
D. a urinalysis should be performed

96. The type of administration that allows the drug the fastest onset of action is
- **A.** intramuscular
- **B.** subcutaneous
- **C.** intravenous
- **D.** sublingual

97. The abbreviation q4h means
- **A.** every 4 days
- **B.** 4 times a day
- **C.** every 4 hours
- **D.** for 4 days

98. Tranquilizers are
- **A.** used in dentistry before root canal therapy
- **B.** used in dentistry after any surgical procedure
- **C.** used in dentistry whenever antibiotics are used
- **D.** almost never used in dentistry

99. The most commonly used analgesic is
- **A.** codeine
- **B.** aspirin
- **C.** meperidine
- **D.** morphine

100. A pulse oximeter measures the arterial blood's
- **A.** O_2 saturation
- **B.** CO_2 saturation
- **C.** pO_2 saturation
- **D.** pCO_2 saturation

101. A drug used to prevent epileptic attacks is
- **A.** ampicillin
- **B.** a tranquilizer
- **C.** Dilantin
- **D.** monoamine oxidase

102. Addictive analgesic drugs are known as
   A. narcotics
   B. antihistamines
   C. tranquilizers
   D. stimulants

103. The function of a hemostatic agent is to
   A. thicken the blood
   B. thin the blood
   C. stop bleeding
   D. increase the number of blood platelets in the circulating blood

104. The most commonly used local anesthetic is
   A. epinephrine
   B. lidocaine (Xylocaine)
   C. Carbocaine
   D. nitrous oxide

105. Epinephrine in local anesthesia causes
   A. increased uptake of the anesthetic by blood vessels
   B. hyperventilation
   C. prolonged effects of the anesthetic
   D. tissue irritation

106. Ethyl chloride can be used as a (an)
   A. topical anesthetic
   B. general anesthetic
   C. inhalant
   D. local anesthetic

107. An antibiotic is a drug
   A. that inhibits viruses
   B. used only for pulmonary infections
   C. that increases circulation
   D. produced by a microorganism that destroys other micro-organisms

108. The use of drugs in cancer therapy is called
   A. radiotherapy
   B. electrocautery

C. chemotherapy

D. psychotherapy

109. The type of drug used for prophylactic premedication for valvular heart disease is
   A. narcotic
   B. antihistamine
   C. antibiotics
   D. tranquilizer

110. A common drug used in the dental office to decrease anxiety is
   A. nitrous oxide
   B. caffeine
   C. aspirin
   D. benzocaine

111. Nitrous oxide should **NOT** be used on patients who have
   A. dental caries
   B. gingival infections
   C. high pain threshold
   D. nasal obstructions

112. A cleft lip is caused by a lack of fusion between the
   A. frontonasal process and median nasal process
   B. maxillary process and median nasal process
   C. maxillary process
   D. soft palate and hard palate

113. All of these are signs of inflammation **EXCEPT**
   A. heat
   B. pain
   C. swelling
   D. regeneration

114. A salivary stone is called
   A. tartar
   B. a salivary nodule
   C. a sialograph
   D. a sialolith

115. Neoplasm refers to
 A. tissue dysplasia
 B. a malignant growth
 C. a new growth
 D. an allergic reaction

DIRECTIONS (Questions 116–130): Match each item in Column A with the appropriate explanation in Column B.

COLUMN A

116. alveolectomy _____
117. excision of
neoplasm _____
118. alveoplasty _____
119. frenectomy _____
120. orthognathic
surgery _____

COLUMN B

A. removal of alveolar bone to eliminate sharp edges of under-cuts
B. reduction and recontouring of the alveolar ridge
C. straightening of the jaws, surgical orthodontics
D. biopsy
E. surgical release of the tissue band inside the lip between the central incisors

COLUMN A

121. preprosthetic
surgery _____
122. sinus lift _____
123. reduction of
fracture _____
124. apicoectomy _____
125. pericoronitis _____

COLUMN B

A. placement of graft material inside the sinus to augment the bony support in the alveolar ridge
B. surgery of soft and hard tissue prior to prosthetic treatment
C. restoration of the bony segments to proper anatomic location
D. inflammation surrounding a partially erupted tooth due to infection
E. surgical removal of the root tip and surrounding bone

COLUMN A

126. incisional biopsy _____
127. excisional biopsy _____
128. alveolitis _____
129. exfoliative cytology_____
130. aspiration biopsy _____

COLUMN B

A. removal of entire lesion including border of normal tissue
around lesion

B. dry socket

C. removal of specific part of a lesion

D. removal of cells by repeated
scraping of lesion

E. removal of fluid with a syringe
and 18-gauge needle

Practice Test Questions 5: Oral and Maxillofacial Surgery

Answers and Discussion

1. **(B)** An impaction is a tooth that will not erupt fully. Most impacted teeth are third molars. These teeth are removed surgically because of pain, to avoid damage to adjacent teeth, or to prevent future complications.

2. **(A)** The basic components of a surgical elevator are the handle, shank, and tip (blade).

3. **(C)** Rongeurs forceps are designed for cutting and contouring bone during a surgical procedure. Rongeurs are shaped as a side or end cutting instrument with spring action handles.

4. **(B)** An instrument that holds a tissue flap away from the operating field is called a retractor. Proper retraction offers the operator better access to and visibility of the surgical site while protecting the flap and surrounding tissue from unnecessary trauma.

5. **(C)** A biopsy is a surgical procedure that removes tissue for diagnostic purposes. There are several types of biopsies: excisional, in which the entire lesion is removed; incisional, in which a wedge-shaped piece of a large lesion is removed; aspiration biopsy, in which a piece of lesion is removed with a large-lumen needle; and exfoliative cytology, in which cells of a lesion are scraped off.

6. (B) Surgical burs are designed with extra long shanks to enable the surgeon to keep the handpiece head in visual field during operational procedures.

7. (B) The basic components of an extraction forcep are the handle, hinge, and beak, which may vary in design. The extraction forcep is used to remove teeth.

8. (C) General anesthetics render patients unconscious by their effect on the central nervous system. These anesthetics can be administered by inhalation or by intravenous injection. The administration of general anesthetics requires special equipment and training and involves a risk that limits its use in the general dental office.

9. (D) Before assisting in surgery in the hospital operating room the assistant should perform a thorough surgical scrub for approximately 10 min. Hands, wrists, and arms to approximately 2″ above the elbow must be cleansed with a surgical scrub soap or solution.

10. (A) Instrument transfer of surgical forceps is done using a two-handed palm grasp.

11. (C)

12. (D)

13. (A)

14. (E)

15. (B)

16. (A) Although monitoring of a patient during surgery is done by the surgical team, the surgeon takes full responsibility for all surgical procedures, including patient monitoring and related complications if they should occur.

17. (C) The body systems monitored during general anesthesia or intravenous sedation are the respiratory system, cardiovascular system, and central nervous system.

18. (C) The pulse is monitored by palpating the radial or carotid arteries with the fingertips.

19. (B) When palpating the pulse you should be aware of the rate, rhythm, and strength of the pulse. The normal rate for an adult is 60 to 100 beats per minute. The rhythm should be constant and regular, with the strength ranging anywhere from very strong to very weak.

20. (A) The characteristics of a laryngospasm are snoring, gurgling, and high-pitched crowing sounds. These sounds indicate that the patient has a partially obstructed airway and immediate emergency treatment must be administered.

21. (D) The electrocardiogram is a graphic tracing of the electrical activity of the heart. The electrocardiogram machine produces the graphic tracing and is used during extensive surgical procedures.

22. (C) After surgery, the patient is instructed not to spit or drink through a straw because this action causes suction and negative pressure in the mouth, resulting in possible bleeding. Postoperative instructions must always be reviewed thoroughly with the patient before beginning surgical procedures.

23. (C) Intravenous barbiturates are classified as sedative-hypnotics. These drugs produce a conscious but sleeplike state.

24. (B) The greatest potential danger of a narcotic analgesic is depression of the respiratory system.

25. (A) Common complications that can be anticipated and prevented during the postoperative recovery period are respiratory obstruction, bodily injury, and hemorrhage. Patients must be monitored closely after surgery to prevent serious postoperative complications.

26. (B) The most common complication associated with implant surgery is the lack of osseointegration, a direct structural and functional connection between living bone and the surface of a dental implant.

27. **(A)** Titanium is a metal that is used for dental implants. Titanium exhibits favorable biomechanical and biocompatible properties.

28. **(C)** Dental implants are classified in the following three categories: endosteal, subperiosteal, and transosteal implants. Endosteal implants (endosseous) are surgically placed within the bone, and transosteal (transosseous) implants are placed through the bone. The subperiosteal dental implant is placed over the bone.

29. **(B)** The most common anesthetic agents used in oral and maxillofacial surgery are Brevital and Diprivan. Both drugs are ultra-short-acting intravenous barbiturates that produce general anesthesia with greater dosages than for sedation.

30. **(D)** Naxolone is one of the most common narcotic antagonists that may be given to reverse the action of a narcotic-based drug.

31. **(C)** The treatment of fractures is the approximation of the parts (reduction) followed by immobilization (fixation) until the bone heals. Reduction can be accomplished by closed reduction, manipulation of the fracture without exposing the bone, or by open reduction, in which the fractured ends of the bones are exposed. Immobilization of the mandible or maxilla is accomplished by wiring the upper and lower teeth together.

32. **(D)** The Caldwell-Luc procedure is performed to remove a displaced tooth in the maxillary sinus.

33. **(B)** Surgical chisels are used in conjunction with a surgical hand mallet to remove bone and split teeth. Some surgical chisels may be driven by a special handpiece.

34. **(A)** The surgical curette is generally used to remove debris, granulomas, and enucleation of small cysts and diseased tissue. The surgical curette also may be used to debride bony tooth sockets after an extraction.

35. **(D)** Elevators are designed in various shapes, sizes, and working angles, and their function is to luxate and remove teeth. The elevator is effective also in the removal of roots and root fragments during surgical procedures.

36. (B) The periosteal elevator is used to reflect the mucoperiosteum and the gingival tissue from around the neck of the tooth before extraction.

37. (D) A drain is a piece of material, usually rubber or gauze, that creates a pathway whereby fluid can leave the body.

38. (A) Before dismissing a patient immediately after surgery, the dental auxiliary must check the patient to see that he or she is not feeling dizzy or experiencing unusual or excessive bleeding. Postoperative instructions must be explained to the patient thoroughly before the surgical procedure begins, and a written copy of the postoperative instructions is given to the patient. If indicated, appropriate arrangements regarding transportation must be made before dismissing the patient if the patient is unable to drive due to medications administered during the surgical procedure. Swelling is a common symptom after any type of surgical procedure and should not present a serious concern.

39. (B) Nitrous oxide is used primarily in oral surgery as an inhalation sedation agent.

40. (A)

41. (C)

42. (B)

43. (D)

44. (B)

45. (A)

46. (C)

47. (B)

48. (A)

49. (D)

50. (B)

51. (A)

52. (C)

53. (B)

54. (A)

55. (B)

56. (A)

57. (C)

58. (B) Health history questionnaires must be completed before rendering clinical dental care. A patient's medical history can affect all phases of a patient's treatment, including prescriptions, preoperative and postoperative instructions, and length of appointments.

59. (C) Universal precautions should be practiced routinely with every patient. All patients are assumed to be able to transmit disease.

60. (B) When taking a blood pressure reading, the first sound heard is recorded as the systolic pressure measurement. Systolic blood pressure is the pressure exerted on the walls of arteries when the heart contracts.

61. (A) The color of the oxygen cylinder tank is always green. Oxygen tanks should be checked periodically to ensure that they are full and functioning properly.

62. (C) The lower edge of the sphygmomanometer cuff should be placed approximately 1″ above the (antecubital fossa) elbow crease. The cuff should be deflated before placement and wrapped evenly and firmly around the arm.

63. (B) The average resting pulse rate for an adult is 60 to 100 heart beats per minute. A normal pulse rate should have a relatively regular rhythm. The pulse rate can increase with exercise and decrease with sleep.

64. (A) The average or normal oral temperature reading for an adult is 98.6° F. Fever is an increase in oral temperature in excess of 101° F.

65. (D) The average respiratory rate for an adult is 16 to 20 breaths per minute.

66. (B) The residual air is the amount of air remaining in the lungs after the deepest exhalation that cannot be expired from the lungs through a voluntary effort. Tidal air is the amount of air that can be handled in a normal inhalation and a normal exhalation.

67. (D) The best way to treat an emergency is to prevent the occurrence of one. The dental assistant must always be alert to any signs or symptoms of impending emergencies that may be exhibited by the dental patient.

68. (B) Short appointments are recommended for patients who have either a physical or mental problem and can be easily stressed by long dental appointments. Patients who have a history of cardiac problems are normally scheduled for shorter dental appointments to avoid undue stress on an already weakened heart.

69. (A) The depressed state of many body functions is called shock. The severity of shock depends on the cause. Some forms of shock are neurogenic, insulin, and anaphylactic.

70. (A) When treating a patient for shock, the victim's feet should be raised 8–12″ above the rest of the body to increase blood circulation in the head.

71. (B) Syncope refers to the lack of blood to the brain for a short period. This is caused by dilation of blood vessels in the body and results in loss of consciousness.

72. (D) Inhalation of spirits of ammonia is used as a reflex stimulant that causes a patient to regain consciousness after fainting. It is stored in individual vials that are broken at the time of use.

73. (B) The treatment for syncope is to place the head lower than the rest of the body, administer aromatic ammonia inhalant, loosen tight clothing, administer oxygen, and give reassurance.

74. (C) Patients with chronic respiratory problems must be positioned in such a manner that may facilitate the breathing process and comfort. In many cases, these patients cannot be placed in a supine position.

75. (D) The proper sequence in an emergency situation is to control severe bleeding, restore breathing, and treat for shock. Only severe bleeding—bleeding that is spurting from a wound as the heart beats—must be controlled immediately. If bleeding is not severe, the immediate priority is to establish an airway.

76. (C) If circulatory collapse occurs, the patient should be given external cardiac massage. This procedure artificially continues the circulation until the patient's heartbeat has been restored or until medical help arrives.

77. (B) Clear foreign matter from the mouth, tilt the head backward with chin pointing up, put one hand on the victim's forehead, and apply firm backward pressure with the palm of the hand to tilt the head back. Place the fingers of the other hand under the bony part of the victim's lower jaw to bring the chin forward, lift the jaw to bring the teeth close together, but do not close the victim's mouth. Pinch the nostrils shut and form a seal over the victim's mouth with your mouth. A disposable microshield may be utilized.

78. (C) Anaphylactic shock is a sudden, violent allergic reaction. Two drugs used in dentistry that may cause this reaction are local anesthesia and penicillin. A detailed, accurate medical history of past adverse drug reactions could indicate whether a drug could cause this reaction.

79. (C) The drug that best counteracts anaphylactic shock is epinephrine; 0.5 mL of 1/1000 epinephrine is injected subcutaneously for this purpose.

80. (B) Patients taking anticoagulation medication must be watched for bleeding problems because this medication diminishes the ability of the blood to clot.

81. (C) Postural hypotension is most likely to occur when the patient's chair position is changed too quickly. Symptoms include lightheadedness, possible loss of consciousness, and low blood pressure. Predisposing factors include patient's taking antihypertensive medications, antidepressants, narcotics, and drugs for Parkinson's disease. To avoid postural hypotension, raise the patient in the dental chair slowly from a supine position to an upright position.

82. (A) The first aid measures that should be rendered to a patient during an epileptic seizure are moving objects away from the patient, loosening the patient's clothing, supporting the patient's breathing if necessary, allowing the patient to rest, and reassuring the patient.

83. (C) During CPR, chest compressions must be given with the victim lying on a firm flat surface. The victim's head should be at the same level as the heart. Begin by locating the lower edge of the victim's ribcage. Gently slide your hand so that the index and middle fingers are placed up the edge of the ribcage to the notch where the ribs meet (the sternum) in the center of the lower part of the chest. The heel of the other hand is placed on the sternum right next to and above the two fingers of the hand resting on the notch.

84. (B) The treatment for an accidentally avulsed central incisor is to rinse the tooth in lukewarm water, reinsert it as soon as possible, and stabilize the reinserted tooth until professional help arrives.

85. (B) Insulin shock results from excess insulin in the blood and can be counteracted by eating a food with high sugar content.

86. (A) Patients with a medical history of diabetes complications should be monitored closely during dental treatment. Medical emergency procedures for a conscious patient undergoing insulin shock include the administration of orange juice, candy, sugar water, soft drinks, or other oral carbohydrates that can easily be made available in the dental office. Office emergency kits should contain packets of sugar if a refrigerator is unavailable to stock other perishable items. The treatment of an unconscious patient in insulin shock requires immediate basic life support procedures and immediate medical attention. Intravenous administration of dextrose usually is required.

87. (D) Patients with a medical history of angina pectoris may be treated with nitroglycerin. Nitroglycerin is a vasodilator and should be administered sublingually for quick onset of the drug. The patient can be made more comfortable by seating in an upright position and administering oxygen if necessary.

88. (E) Lawsuits can be avoided by keeping accurate records and completely documenting all dental procedures rendered. Entries must be made in ink, and medical health histories must be updated periodically. Appropriate patient treatment consent forms must be signed and on file in case of a potential lawsuit. Each state sets certain standards and limitations regarding dental assistant procedures that must be adhered to strictly in order to remain within the defined legal boundaries of the state Dental Practice Act.

89. (D) The human brain requires oxygen to function. Without oxygen, a state of unconsciousness will occur rapidly. In emergency situations where airway obstruction exists, permanent brain damage (brain cell death) will occur within 4–6 min.

90. (D) Symptoms of diabetic coma (ketoacidosis) include weak pulse, low blood pressure, dry mouth and thirst, flushed skin tone, confusion, general weakness or drowsiness, and acetone breath odor. Diabetic coma may occur from an insufficient amount of insulin or failure to take insulin medication when indicated.

91. (B) Medical emergency treatment for the patient who is experiencing hyperventilation includes reassuring and calming the patient and having the patient take several deep slow breaths. A paper bag may be held gently over the patient's mouth and nose to correct the hyperventilation syndrome by having the patient breathe in his or her own exhaled air, which contains carbon dioxide.

92. **(A)** Cerebrovascular accident (CVA) is also known as a stroke. A CVA is caused by a sudden loss of brain function due to an interruption of the blood supply to the brain. Symptoms of CVA may include an irregular or thready pulse, slurred speech, dilated pupils, slow labored breathing, and cyanosis (bluish discoloration of the skin).

93. **(E)** A basic office emergency armamentarium includes intravenous armamentarium and related drugs, sponges, tourniquets, syringes, mouth props, and sugar packs. A portable oxygen tank also is considered a basic necessity of the medical emergency kit.

94. **(D)** The patient with a history of liver disease (hepatitis) should be given limited quantities of local anesthetic. Liver damage may indicate difficulty in metabolizing the injected anesthetic drug, causing an elevated anesthetic level in the patient's blood.

95. **(A)** Before prescribing any drug, an accurate medical history must be taken. Some factors in a patient's history that can influence drug administration are a history of drug allergies, other drugs the patient might be taking, and physical and mental states.

96. **(C)** Intravenous drug administration has the fastest onset of action. An intravenous injection introduces the drug directly into the bloodstream. This method is also used to infuse a large amount of fluid into the body.

97. **(C)** Some common Latin abbreviations are q4h (every 4 hours), qid (4 times a day), prn (as needed), and ac (before meals).

98. **(D)** Tranquilizers are rarely used in dentistry. These drugs are used for their long-range sedating effects.

99. **(B)** The most commonly used analgesic is aspirin. Aspirin also functions as an antirheumatic, antipyretic, and antiinflammatory agent.

100. (A) A pulse oximeter is a machine with a finger probe that reads the blood pulsating through the finger and determines the level of oxygen saturated hemoglobin. Normal levels are between 95% and 99%.

101. (C) A drug used to prevent epileptic attacks is diphenylhydantoin (Dilantin). A side effect of this drug is fibrous hyperplasia of the gingiva.

102. (A) Addictive analgesic drugs are narcotics. Care must be taken when these drugs are prescribed, since they can become physiologically habit forming.

103. (C) Hemostatic agents stop bleeding by aiding the normal clotting mechanism. Examples of hemostatic agents used in dentistry are absorbable gelatin sponges, absorbable oxidized cellulose, and alum.

104. (B) The most commonly used local anesthetic is lidocaine (Xylocaine). Local anesthetics can be classified into four groups: para-aminobenzoic acid, meta-aminobenzoic acid, benzoic acid, and amides.

105. (C) Epinephrine in local anesthesia causes prolonged effects of anesthesia. Epinephrine is a vasoconstrictor. It decreases the size of the blood vessels, resulting in a decrease of the circulation in the area, and the anesthetic remains active for a longer period of time.

106. (A) Ethyl chloride can be used as a topical anesthetic. Ethyl chloride temporarily freezes the area to which it is applied.

107. (D) An antibiotic is a drug produced by a microorganism that destroys bacteria. Commonly used antibiotics are penicillin, erythromycin, tetracycline, streptomycin, bacitracin, and chloramphenicol.

108. (C) The use of drugs in cancer therapy is called chemotherapy. Other modes of treatment for cancer are surgery and radiation.

109. (C) Prophylactic means preventing disease. Examples of prophylactic measures are the use of antibiotics to prevent subacute bacterial endocarditis (SBE) or infective endocarditis. Infective endocarditis is a microbial (bacterial) infection of the heart valves that have been damaged in a previous episode of rheumatic fever or rheumatic heart disease. Antibiotic premedication is also required for patients with a history of reduced capacity to resist infection, prosthetic heart valves, mitral valve prolapse, renal transplant or dialysis, and prosthetic joint replacements of the body.

110. (A) Nitrous oxide-oxygen often is used as a sedative in the dental office. It is applied to a patient through a nose mask. The sedative effects are eliminated at the end of the procedure by giving the patient pure oxygen.

111. (D) Nitrous oxide should not be used on patients with nasal obstructions, since the drug is an inhalation agent and is ineffective if not inhaled sufficiently. Patients with other nasal complications, such as sinusitis or nasal injuries, preventing proper inhalation methods are not good candidates for the administration of nitrous oxide.

112. (B) A cleft lip is a defect below the ala of the nose on one or both sides. It is caused by the lack of fusion between the maxillary process and the median nasal process. A cleft palate is the lack of fusion along the medial line of the palate. It can vary from a cleft of part of the soft palate to a cleft of the entire soft and hard palate.

113. (D) Symptoms of inflammation are redness, heat, swelling, and pain. Regeneration is not a sign of the inflammation process.

114. (D) A salivary stone is known as a sialolith. If the stone blocks the duct of a salivary gland, the gland may swell due to the back-up of saliva. Treatment is removal of the stone by manipulation or surgery.

115. (C) Neoplasm refers to a new growth that will not disappear when the etiologic agent is removed. Neoplasms are classified as benign or malignant. Malignant tumors are life threatening and will result in the death of the host if they are not removed.

116. **(A)**

117. **(D)**

118. **(B)**

119. **(E)**

120. **(C)**

121. **(B)**

122. **(A)**

123. **(C)**

124. **(E)**

125. **(D)**

126. **(C)**

127. **(A)**

128. **(B)**

129. **(D)**

130. **(E)**

Practice Test Questions 6: Dental Practice Management

DIRECTIONS (Questions 1–60): Each of the questions or incomplete statements in this section is followed by four suggested answers or completions. Select the **ONE** lettered answer or completion that is **BEST** in each case.

---

1. Ethics refers to
   A. accreditation by the American Dental Association
   B. professional standards of conduct
   C. jurisprudence
   D. membership in the American Dental Assistants Association

2. What determines which duties the dental assistant can perform?
   A. State law
   B. Federal law
   C. Common law
   D. The dentist

3. Who is responsible for duties delegated to assistants?
   A. The receptionist
   B. The office manager
   C. The dentist
   D. The patient

4. The period of time in which a patient may bring suit against a dentist is known as
   A. probationary time
   B. libel
   C. tort
   D. statute of limitations

5. A patient suing for malpractice may include in the suit
   A. the dental assistant
   B. the dentist only
   C. the hygienist and dentist only
   D. anyone working in the dental practice

6. Patient records are
   A. public information
   B. available only to relatives
   C. confidential records and private property
   D. released at the assistant's discretion

7. An appropriate response when answering the phone is
   A. "This is Dr. Smith's office. Pat Jones speaking. May I help you?"
   B. "Who's calling?"
   C. "With whom would you like to speak?"
   D. "May I help you?"

8. A patient calls and complains about the treatment given. The receptionist should
   A. justify the dentist's position
   B. engage in a verbal duel
   C. take the patient's side
   D. allow the dentist to handle the situation

9. A telephone caller asks the price of a full mouth rehabilitation. The receptionist should
   A. estimate the price
   B. ask the patient to come in for an examination
   C. put the dentist on the phone to quote prices
   D. refer the person elsewhere

10. What is a contract?
   A. An analysis of assets against liabilities
   B. An agreement between two or more people
   C. Records of work completed
   D. An unexpected action

11. A case presentation is a
   A. treatment conference with the patient
   B. case that is sent to the laboratory for construction
   C. paper or speech presented by the doctor to a dental society
   D. study model used to diagnose a case

12. Which person traditionally controls the appointment book?
   A. Dentist
   B. Chairside assistant
   C. Receptionist
   D. Hygienist

13. An office manual is
   A. a procedural guide for all office activities
   B. detailed information on how the equipment should be serviced
   C. the doctor's instructions for operating equipment most efficiently
   D. the record that the business assistant keeps for the accountant

14. Overhead is
   A. net income
   B. the cost necessary to practice dentistry
   C. assets of the practice
   D. the break-even production point

15. The money paid to the dental practice is known as its
   A. gross income
   B. liabilities
   C. net income
   D. expenses

16. A day sheet in each treatment room provides which of the following data?
  A. Any serious medical problem that could affect treatment
  B. The patient's occupation
  C. The procedure to be performed and length of the appointment
  D. The number of visits needed to complete treatment

17. Mr. Jones completed his dental treatment in September. For a 6-month recall he should return in
  A. January
  B. March
  C. April
  D. June

18. Under the OSHA (Occupational Safety Health Administration) standard the records of an employee's exposure incident are to be
  A. entered into the office computer data bank for easy access
  B. kept confidential and filed in the employee's medical record
  C. faxed to the employee's private physician
  D. kept on file for 1 full year

19. A list of equipment and supplies present in the office is known as
  A. expendables
  B. overhead
  C. the office manual
  D. an inventory

20. An invoice is a
  A. statement of money collected
  B. bill for items shipped
  C. cash receipt
  D. form of vertical filing

21. When generating and processing electronic insurance claims through the office computer system it is necessary to
  A. log the information into the daily appointment schedule
  B. enter the information onto a deposit slip
  C. keep a back-up file and paper record of claim
  D. mail a copy to the insurance company

22. Postoperative telephone calls are necessary for all of the following **EXCEPT**
    A. to remind patients of postoperative care they should be carrying out
    B. to remind patients of their appointments for postoperative treatment
    C. to show patients special concern
    D. to discuss the patient's payment schedule

23. An effective method to ensure that the patient will keep an appointment made over the telephone is to
    A. overlap appointments
    B. charge the patient for missed appointments
    C. send a written confirmation
    D. repeat the appointment time before hanging up

24. Factors to be considered in appointment scheduling include all of the following **EXCEPT**
    A. the emergency patient
    B. management of prime time
    C. young children or elderly patients
    D. the business assistant's lunch time

25. A patient requires several appointments, each a week apart. The best scheduling would be to assign the patient
    A. the same time and day each week
    B. randomly
    C. Monday the first week, Tuesday the second week, Wednesday the next week, and so forth
    D. relative to the payment arrangements

26. Which of the following statements is **NOT** true about double-entry bookkeeping?
    A. It clearly shows both the debit and credit for every office transaction
    B. It provides the necessary components to balance books
    C. It assists the dentist in determining fees
    D. It provides a record if a patient's payment card is lost or misplaced

27. Third party refers to
   A. children of patients
   B. insurance carriers
   C. a group of general dentists and specialists
   D. patients receiving public assistance

28. Insurance forms should always be
   A. accompanied by x-ray films
   B. accompanied by study models
   C. duplicated for office records
   D. mailed first class

29. A truth-in-lending form is
   A. a contract signed by the patient
   B. a contract signed by the doctor
   C. a government requirement to protect all patients who pay for treatment in advance
   D. a government requirement to protect patients from hidden finance charges in installment payments

30. Dental records
   A. are not admissible as evidence
   B. should always be typed
   C. are legally admissible as evidence
   D. minimize a dentist's risk of liability if filled out in ink

31. What records are kept in an inactive file?
   A. Records of all patients who have completed treatment
   B. Records of patients who will return in 1 year
   C. Records of patients no longer seeking treatment at the office
   D. Records of patients who receive treatment at a discount

32. Accounts receivable are
   A. monies owed to the dentist from insurance carriers
   B. all monies owed to the dentist for completed treatment
   C. all monies that the dentist owes to creditors
   D. all monies owed to the dentist for future treatment

33. As accounts receivable age, they
   A. increase in value
   B. remain the same in value
   C. decrease in value
   D. are placed in an inactive file

34. Capitation programs are widely used in
   A. PPOs (Preferred Provider Organizations)
   B. IPAs (Individual Practice Associations)
   C. DRPs (Direct Reimbursement Plans)
   D. HMOs (Health Maintenance Organizations)

35. Third-party precertification (or prior authorization) will inform the
   A. dentist and patient of the obligation assumed by the third party
   B. dentist of the correct treatment plan
   C. dentist that prepayment is available
   D. patient of the dentist's skills

36. A patient denies payment responsibilities. The next course of action is
   A. to forget about the bill
   B. to contact a collection agency
   C. harassment
   D. to notify the patient's employer

37. Insurance codes and nomenclature for specific dental treatment procedures are obtained in the
   A. CDT published by the American Dental Association
   B. CDC (Centers for Disease Control) publication
   C. third-party carrier's manual
   D. office procedures manual

38. Federal regulations that affect the practice of dentistry regarding "public accommodations" include the
   A. Occupational Safety Health Administration (OSHA) regulations
   B. Environmental Protection Agency (EPA) regulations
   C. Internal Revenue Service (IRS) regulations
   D. Americans with Disabilities Act (ADA)-Title III regulations

39. When you go through the appointment book and block off time, such as staff meetings, this is called
   A. deleting
   B. outlining
   C. scheduling
   D. confirming

40. If patients are habitually late, the assistant should
   A. not give them another appointment
   B. give them a stern lecture on the importance of being on time
   C. schedule their appointments in your appointment book 15 min. after the time you listed on their appointment cards
   D. inform them later of an extra charge

41. The Certified Dental Assistant may dispense medication to the patient
   A. after oral surgery
   B. by checking labels and amount of drugs
   C. after checking for allergies the patient may have
   D. under direct supervision of the dentist

42. All insurance carriers use
   A. the same table of benefits
   B. different tables of benefits depending on the type of coverage to which the subscriber is entitled
   C. a percentage of the dentist's usual and customary fees
   D. closed-panel dental care for their subscribers

43. Which of the following OSHA (Occupational Safety and Health Administration) requirements must the employer provide in order to ensure safe work practices for the employees?
   A. Post emergency exit signs and provide fire extinguishers
   B. Hold periodic staff meetings
   C. Invite OSHA inspectors for office tours
   D. Provide lead-lined aprons and thyroid collars for patients

44. When a patient calls and insists on speaking to the doctor, the assistant should
   A. call the doctor to the phone as promptly as possible
   B. explain to the patient that it is the responsibility of the assistant to respond to phone calls

    C. explain that the doctor is treating a patient and that he or she will return the call as soon as possible

    D. tell the patient to call back at a specific hour

45. Assignment of benefits means that

    A. the patient is entitled to complete reimbursement for his or her dental care in each given year

    B. the dentist receives direct payment from the insurance carrier in the amount that the patient's insurance plan designates

    C. all members of the immediate family of the insured are entitled to insurance coverage in a given year

    D. if a patient does not use insurance benefits in a given year, he or she can allot these benefits to an immediate family member

46. A patient cancels an appointment an hour before he is due. A good course of action is to

    A. close the office at the appointment time

    B. allow the dentist to resolve the problem

    C. call a patient who is available on short notice

    D. announce a coffee break to the dentist and rest of the staff

47. The rights of a patient during the treatment phase do **NOT** include

    A. the right to be informed about his or her condition

    B. the right to refuse treatment

    C. the right to confidential records

    D. the right to dictate the course of treatment

48. Cross-training means

    A. assistants are knowledgeable about each other's jobs

    B. dental assistants can perform some of the procedures usually delegated to the hygienists

    C. assistants are trained in a school environment

    D. assistants receive on-the-job training

49. Every dental office is required to maintain a written hazard communication program which contains all of the following **EXCEPT**

    A. material safety data sheets (MSDS)

    B. laundry schedules and costs

    C. hazardous chemicals log

    D. employee training records for Hazard Communication Standard

50. A bank statement will show which of the following?
   A. Only deposits made
   B. The customer's credit account
   C. Checks paid, deposits, and the balance
   D. Customer credit card charges

51. The patient's name should be entered in the appointment book
   A. before the day's treatment is complete
   B. after mailing the recall appointment
   C. when the appointment is made
   D. after the appointment is completed

52. When a patient suffering pain of dental origin calls for an appointment, the assistant should
   A. have the patient come in immediately for temporary relief
   B. make an appointment for next week
   C. make an appointment the following day
   D. refer to another dentist

53. Net pay refers to
   A. salary after deductions
   B. total collections minus office expense
   C. taxable wages plus tips
   D. total amount used to figure payroll taxes

54. Gross pay refers to
   A. total collections of accounts receivable per month
   B. salary after deductions
   C. salary before deductions
   D. total collections minus office expenses

55. Which of the following taxes is **NOT** a payroll tax?
   A. State Disability Insurance
   B. Social Security
   C. Federal Income Tax
   D. Federal Excise Tax

56. A recall system based on making advance appointments is called
    A. standby appointments
    B. continuing appointments
    C. chronologic file system
    D. instant reference system

57. In the filing rule regarding surname, the correct indexing order is
    A. first name, middle name, surname
    B. surname, first name, middle name
    C. middle name, first name, surname
    D. surname, middle name, first name

58. The most frequently used adult charting system is to
    A. number the teeth from 1–32 beginning with the maxillary right third molar
    B. number the teeth in each quadrant from 1–8 beginning with third molars
    C. number the teeth in each quadrant from 1–8 beginning with central incisors
    D. letter the teeth beginning with the maxillary right third molar

59. UCR stands for
    A. unusual, coverage, regular
    B. usual, carrier, reasonable
    C. usual, customary, reasonable
    D. usual, claim, rider

60. When storing supplies, you should
    A. store frequently used items in an easily accessible area
    B. store frequently used items out of reach
    C. store film near a heat source
    D. store cements in the refrigerator

DIRECTIONS: (Questions 61–65): Match the items in Column A with the appropriate definition in Column B.

COLUMN A

61. alphabetizing _____
62. copayment _____
63. authorization to release information _____
64. filing _____
65. carrier _____

COLUMN B

A. the patient's signature giving consent for the release of information relative to his or her claim

B. the act of classifying and arranging records so they will be preserved safely and in such a manner that records can be retrieved easily

C. an arrangement under which the carrier and beneficiary are each responsible for a fixed share of the cost of dental services

D. the arrangement of captions and indexing units in strict alphabetical order

E. the insurance company or dental plan that agrees to pay the benefits

---

DIRECTIONS (Questions 66–79): Each of the questions or incomplete statements in this section is followed by four suggested answers or completions. Select the **ONE** lettered answer or completion that is **BEST** in each case.

---

66. Necessary information required for the patient account record includes all of the following **EXCEPT**
  A. home telephone number
  B. home address
  C. name and address of employer
  D. hours worked each week

67. A treatment plan is a (an)
    A. approach to collections
    B. inventory control system
    C. peer evaluation system
    D. systematic approach to meet the dental needs of the patient

68. A running inventory is
    A. a system of altering the supply list to know which supplies are present in the office
    B. moving the inventory from place to place
    C. a billing technique
    D. an inventory updated once a year

69. The main advantage of purchasing a large quantity of a particular supply at one time is
    A. it is easy to store
    B. to save money when buying in bulk
    C. the billing is easier
    D. the dental materials have an indefinite shelf life

70. When recalling patients by telephone, the business assistant should
    A. call early in the day
    B. leave a message on the answering machine
    C. insist that the patient commit to a specific time
    D. have the patient's recall record ready for reference

71. All fees charged and payments received should be entered promptly on the daily journal page and
    A. patient ledger card
    B. charge slip
    C. receipts
    D. appointment book

72. An office manual is most effective when it is
    A. purchased from a reputable dental supply company
    B. organized by a professional management consultant who has evaluated the practice
    C. organized by the dentist and the staff in keeping with the office's philosophy, goals, and objectives
    D. a collection of directions that the dentist believes is appropriate for his or her mode of dental care delivery

73. Pegboard accounting materials include all of the following **EXCEPT**
    A. receipts and charge slips
    B. ledgers
    C. daily journal page
    D. bank deposit slips

74. Which of the following does **NOT** describe an active file?
    A. Waiting insurance approval
    B. Patient under treatment
    C. Treatment complete but with balance
    D. Treatment completed and paid

75. Mark Jones received the following dental treatment: an examination and x-rays ($25), five surfaces of amalgam restorations (at $8 per surface), and two extractions (at $10 per extraction). The total fee for his dental treatment is
    A. $85
    B. $43
    C. $75
    D. $77

76. When filling out a deposit slip, the auxiliary must
    A. not endorse the checks before depositing
    B. list checks and currency separately
    C. only list deposits over $100
    D. list all checks in alphabetical order

77. When a check from a patient has been returned, it is best to
    A. immediately send the patient to collections
    B. convert the missing money from petty cash
    C. adjust the balance of the patient's account accordingly
    D. ask patient to initiate a stop payment order

78. With reference to a stop payment order on checks, all of the following are true **EXCEPT**
    A. the stop payment indicates insufficient funds
    B. the stop payment order may be made by phone
    C. the stop payment order may be made by filling out proper bank forms at the bank
    D. payment can be stopped if there is reason to believe the check has been lost

79. To double check entries on the daily journal record and patient ledger cards to ensure that all entries and calculations are accurate refers to
   A. proof-of-posting
   B. monthly summary
   C. cross-reference
   D. computer processing

DIRECTIONS (Questions 80–85): Refer to Figure 6–1 to answer Questions 80 through 85.

---

80. The bank deposit for this day is
   A. $100
   B. $192
   C. $275
   D. $375

81. The total for column A is
   A. $275
   B. $375
   C. $534
   D. $540

PROFESSIONAL SERVICE	A CHARGE	B PAID	C NEW BALANCE	D PREVIOUS BALANCE	NAME
BALANCE FWD.					
Ex,X,P. (ck)	30 00	30 00	—	—	Mary Knight
SR.	24 00	—	36 00	12 00	Lisa Daniels
G.T. (a)	16 00	28 00	—	12 00	Robert Smith
Ex, X, D.S.(ck)	89 00	34 00	55 00	—	Charles Johnson
C&B (ck)	375 00	100 00	275 00	—	Harold Turner

SHEET NO. ____

PROOF OF POSTING

Figure 6–1

82. The total for column C is
A. $275
B. $366
C. $375
D. $396

83. The total for column B is
A. $100
B. $175
C. $192
D. $292

84. The total for column D is
A. $12
B. $21
C. $23
D. $24

85. To perform proof-of-posting properly, the subtotal for column D plus column A would be
A. $534
B. $558
C. $366
D. $24

DIRECTIONS (Questions 86–100): Each of the questions or incomplete statements in this section is followed by four suggested answers or completions. Select the **ONE** lettered answer or completion that is **BEST** in each case.

---

86. The office manual includes all of the following **EXCEPT**
A. statement of purpose or objectives
B. staff policies
C. medical emergency procedures
D. payroll records

87. When a patient is injured by a dentist's employee
A. the dentist is not liable
B. the employee is the only one who can be sued by the patient
C. the employee is not liable
D. the employee and dentist are both liable

88. Things to avoid during an interview include all of the following **EXCEPT**
   A. chewing gum
   B. lacking a neat appearance
   C. using eye contact
   D. talking about salary and hours immediately

89. Consent to an operation or to a course of treatment
   A. must be actual only
   B. is a professional duty to the public
   C. is not necessary for the dentist to obtain
   D. may be expressed or implied

90. Anything done to a person without consent is
   A. a skill and judgment
   B. a judgment
   C. a trespass
   D. proof of freedom from contributory negligence

91. Written records on patients kept by the dentist
   A. are of little value in malpractice cases
   B. should always be filled in erasable ink
   C. make up the single most important factor in the defense of most malpractice cases
   D. make expert testimony unnecessary

92. Professional liability claims are most likely to be based on
   A. the charge of a faulty patient medical history
   B. the charge of faulty patient x-rays
   C. the charge of faulty or erroneous diagnosis
   D. the charge of faulty dental equipment

93. Negligence is
   A. a legal duty to the public
   B. a general duty to the dental profession
   C. a general duty to the legal profession
   D. the failure to exercise reasonable and ordinary care to avoid injury to others

94. Supplies can be divided into all of the following categories **EXCEPT**
   A. capital items
   B. expendable items
   C. nonexpendable items
   D. receivables

95. The most acceptable payment arrangements in a dental office include all of the following **EXCEPT**
   A. open accounts
   B. advance payments
   C. fixed amount each visit
   D. divided payments

96. Canceled checks
   A. are never enclosed with a monthly bank statement
   B. are the same as voided checks
   C. should be credited to the account
   D. have been paid and charged to the depositor's account

97. Which of the following is true in reference to petty cash?
   A. It is money to pay for inexpensive office items
   B. It is the same as the Christmas fund
   C. A $50 check is written every 6 months to replenish
   D. The cash can be used by the doctor for office uniforms

98. A cashier's check
   A. is also called a certified check
   B. is a bank's own check drawn on itself
   C. is the same as a canceled check
   D. need not be endorsed

99. Which of the following steps is **NOT** included in the bank reconciliation procedure?
   A. Compare canceled checks to bank statement
   B. Calculate deposits in transit
   C. List outstanding checks
   D. Subtract bank service charges from the bank statement total

100. Responsibilities of the business assistant may include which of the following?

   A. Exposing x-rays
   B. Assisting in operative procedures
   C. Interviewing and training new employees
   D. Keeping the treatment area updated with supplies

DIRECTIONS (Questions 101–104): For each of the items in this section, **ONE** or **MORE** of the numbered options is correct. Choose answer

   A. if only 1, 2, and 3 are correct
   B. if only 1 and 3 are correct
   C. if only 2 and 4 are correct
   D. if only 4 is correct
   E. if all are correct

---

101. If a patient presents inappropriate behavior while in the patient reception area, the business assistant should

   1. ask the chairside assistant to seat the patient immediately
   2. allow the patient to continue disrupting the other patients
   3. refer the patient to another office
   4. speak directly to the patient in a firm but professional manner

102. Appointment control will

   1. prevent faulty dentistry
   2. organize the doctor's production time
   3. prevent emergency patients
   4. keep hours within desired limits

103. Record keeping

   1. provides production records
   2. provides a history of treatment success or failure
   3. is needed legally to avoid possible malpractice involvement
   4. avoids the need of an accountant

104. During an office medical emergency situation, the business assistant should

   1. assist the doctor and chairside assistant where needed
   2. update the patient's health history form
   3. call for emergency medical support personnel
   4. administer CPR immediately to the patient

Practice Test Questions 6: Dental Practice Management

Answers and Discussion

1. **(B)** Ethics is the moral obligation that dictates the standards of conduct expected by the dental profession. The ADAA has a written code of ethics to which the assistant is expected to adhere.

2. **(A)** The various state Dental Practice Acts determine which duties the dental assistant can perform. These laws, as all laws, are subject to change, and many have been revised recently to expand the duties of assistants.

3. **(C)** The dentist is responsible for duties delegated to assistants on his or her dental team. He or she must supervise the performance of these duties and ensure the quality of the final product.

4. **(D)** The statute of limitations specifies a period of time in which a patient may bring suit against a dentist. This time varies according to many factors, such as the age of the patient and the reason for the suit.

5. **(D)** A patient suing for malpractice may include in the suit anyone working in the dental practice. Under the principle of respon-

deat superior, "Let the higher one answer," the dentist (employer) is ultimately responsible for the wrongful acts of the staff (agents) while such acts are performed within the employment setting of the employer. Each individual employee may be named in a lawsuit and should individually carry personal liability insurance.

6. **(C)** Patient records are a confidential written history of financial and treatment experiences. These records should not be released or made public without the permission of the patient. Records include dental treatment plan, x-rays, study models, charting records, insurance records, and financial statements.

7. **(A)** An excellent response when answering the phone is, "This is Dr. Smith's office. Pat Jones speaking. May I help you?" The most important part of this communication is the identification of the office.

8. **(D)** The receptionist should allow the dentist to resolve patient problems dealing with the patient's dissatisfaction with treatment. Technical explanations are often required, which are the responsibility of the dentist.

9. **(B)** Fees have many contingencies that cannot be determined over the telephone. Therefore, patients seeking fee quotations should be scheduled for examination.

10. **(B)** A contract is a legal agreement between two or more people. Contracts may be explicit (verbal or written) or implicit (implied, not explicitly expressed). Examples of dental contracts are schedule arrangements, payment arrangements, and job duties.

11. **(A)** The case presentation is the treatment conference where the dentist explains to the patient the findings of the examination and discusses what treatment procedures are necessary in order to restore the patient's mouth to optimum oral health.

12. **(C)** One person should control the appointment book at all times. It is usually the receptionist in an office where several assistants are employed.

13. **(A)** Every office should have a current manual that details all office tasks, policies, and procedures, in addition to goals, objectives, and philosophy of practice.

14. **(B)** Overhead is the cost needed to produce dentistry. It includes rent, supplies, and salaries.

15. **(A)** The money paid to the dental practice is its gross income. The gross income minus the overhead results in the net income.

16. **(C)** A day sheet provides the dentist and office staff with the day's procedures and the length of each appointment.

17. **(B)** A patient who has completed dental treatment in September and is placed on a 6-month recall will be rescheduled in March.

18. **(B)** The records of an employee's exposure incident are to be kept in a confidential employee medical record file. The employer is responsible for the file, which must be retained for the duration of an employee's employment plus 30 years.

19. **(D)** A list of equipment and supplies on hand is known as an inventory. One person in the office should be responsible for maintaining the inventory.

20. **(B)** An invoice is an itemized bill of supplies sent to the dentist. Before paying this bill, the invoice should be checked against the supplies received.

21. **(C)** When generating and processing electronic insurance claims it is necessary to keep a back-up file of the claim in the computer. A paper record is also recommended for tracking purposes in the event that the computer information is deleted.

22. **(D)** Postoperative calls usually are made at the end of the day to patients who have had difficult procedures performed. The rationale for these calls is to show the patients concern, to remind patients of their postoperative responsibilities (e.g., taking medications, rinsing), and to remind them of their next appointment.

23. (C) To ensure that the patient will keep an appointment made over the telephone, the receptionist should send a written confirmation.

24. (D) Although it is necessary for the business assistant to have a lunch break, this is not considered a prime factor in appointment scheduling. The patient always comes first.

25. (A) A patient needing a series of visits should be given appointments at the same time and day each week. This pattern helps the patient remember the appointments.

26. (C) Fees are determined by a careful analysis of expenses (e.g., office overhead). The purpose of a double-entry bookkeeping system is to record income (both collected and outstanding).

27. (B) In a dental office, third party refers to an insurance carrier. All money paid by a particular insurance company is known as third-party payment.

28. (C) Insurance forms, records, x-ray films, study models, and other items that leave the office for any reason should be duplicated in case of loss.

29. (D) Any office that makes arrangements for patients to pay for their dentistry via installments is required by law to provide the patient with a truth-in-lending form. This form indicates whether or not a finance charge will be added if there is a default on payment.

30. (C) Dental records are often the most important pieces of evidence in court and are legally admissible as evidence. Records must always be kept updated, and all entries must be made in ink. Radiographs and models may be included as part of the dental treatment record and should be properly labeled, including patient name and date.

31. (C) The two patient records that are filed as active or inactive are treatment and financial records. The treatment record is placed in an inactive file if the patient is no longer seeking care at the office. The financial record is placed in an inactive file if the account has been fully paid.

32. (B) All unpaid charges for treatment that has been completed are considered accounts receivable.

33. (C) As accounts receivable age, they decrease in value and become more difficult to collect. Therefore, firm payment arrangements are a necessity for a successful practice.

34. (D) Capitation programs include HMOs. Under capitation the dentist has contracted to provide dental services to subscribers for payment on a per capita basis.

35. (A) Third-party precertification will inform the dentist and patient of the obligation assumed by the third party. The money allocated by the insurance company is usually partial payment and is given to the patient or dentist after treatment is completed.

36. (B) Each office has a policy about payment. If a patient has had dental work completed and then denies payment responsibility, the dentist usually will contact a collection agency to begin appropriate legal action.

37. (A) The CDT (Current Dental Terminology) publication from the American Dental Association provides information on nomenclature and appropriate dental procedure codes.

38. (D) Title III of the Americans with Disabilities Act has specific regulations for all dental practices. The ADA requires dentists to make reasonable accommodations in their offices to facilitate access by disabled individuals. Examples of accommodations may include designating parking spaces for the disabled and widening doorways for wheelchair access.

39. (B) Outlining the appointment book designates what time periods the office is closed, such as days off, lunch time, holidays, and vacation time. Outlining the appointment book also indicates blocks of time per day that have been set aside to handle emergency appointments or staff meetings.

40. (C) A good procedure to follow to ensure that a habitually late patient will arrive on time is to schedule the appointment in the book 15 min. after the time listed on the patient's appointment card.

41. (D) The Certified Dental Assistant may dispense medication to the patient under the direct supervision of the dentist only. All medications dispensed to the patient must be documented in the patient dental record, including date, name of drug, and amount dispensed. If an office drug log is kept, the dispensed medication must be recorded and initialed by 2 staff members.

42. (B) It is important that benefits be determined before treatment begins and that the patient be made aware of how much (or little) he or she might receive from the insurance company.

43. (A) OSHA regulations state that the dental employer must provide a fire-safety policy including the training of employees in the use of a fire extinguisher. A diagram of the office layout including emergency exits and the location of all fire extinguishers in the office is required. Emergency phone numbers for ambulance, fire, and police services must be posted.

44. (C) In an effort to conserve the doctor's time and also permit him or her to provide the appropriate attention to the patient in the chair, the business assistant should make every effort to cope with all telephone calls. In those situations when it is necessary for the patient to speak to the doctor, the assistant should explain that the doctor will return the call as soon as possible. It is then the assistant's responsibility to see that the message is given to the doctor.

45. (B) The dental office that accepts assignment of benefits must be sure the patient signs the portion of the insurance form that indicates the money should be sent directly to the dentist. This is done before treatment commences.

46. (C) A cancellation close to the appointed time can be handled by calling a patient who is available on short notice, by extending the visit of the patient who is present before the cancellation, or by moving a patient to be seen later in the day into the time slot.

47. (D) Although patients have many rights pertaining to professional care, the right to determine the proper course of treatment belongs to the dentist.

48. (A) It is important for every dental assistant to be aware of his or her own job description and be capable of fulfilling those specific tasks in the most efficient manner. A dental assistant who is cross-trained also has a working knowledge about the procedures assigned to other assistants and is capable of performing those tasks should it become necessary in time of absence or during a particularly busy period.

49. (B) Laundry schedules and the office costs for laundry service are not part of the OSHA written hazard communication program.

50. (C) A bank statement is issued by the bank and is a record of all transactions, including deposits, withdrawals, canceled checks, and the existing balance. Bank statements usually cover a specific time period and may be calculated on a monthly basis.

51. (C) The patient's complete name, telephone number (home or work), and type of treatment to be rendered must be entered legibly in the appointment book. All appointment book entries should be made in pencil and be erasable in case of a change. In order to minimize appointment errors, it is best to enter this information in the appointment book at the time that the appointment is being made. The appointment card should be completed after the appointment book entry is made. It is best to confirm by phone all appointments made through the mail before entering the name in the appointment book.

52. (A) When a patient suffering from pain of dental origin calls for an appointment, the dental assistant should obtain basic information regarding the nature of the pain, such as duration of pain, which tooth or area is involved, or if there has been a traumatic injury to the area. This basic information will assist the doctor and chairside assistant in preparing for the emergency appointment. The patient should be given an immediate appointment for temporary relief.

53. (A) Net pay refers to salary earned after deductions. The net pay plus all deductions will equal the gross pay.

54. (C) Gross pay refers to the total amount earned before deductions, or the gross salary earnings.

55. (D) Federal law requires that Social Security Tax and Federal Income Tax (withholding) be withheld from each employee. Most states also require withholding of state tax, such as State Disability. Federal Excise Tax is not a payroll tax. It is a separate operational fee that must be paid by the business owner to operate the place of business. The Federal Excise Tax is assessed and collected by the Federal government.

56. (B) A recall system based on making advance appointments is known as a continuing appointment system.

57. (B) In the filing rule regarding surname, the correct indexing order is surname (last name), given name (first name), and middle name or middle initial.

58. (A) The most frequently used adult charting system is the universal numbering system, which numbers the teeth from 1 through 32, starting with the maxillary right third molar, which is numbered 1, and continuing across to the maxillary left third molar, which is numbered 16. The mandibular left third molar is numbered 17, and the numbering continues across to the mandibular right third molar, which is numbered 32.

59. (C) The abbreviation UCR is associated with the dental insurance fee-for-service concept. A method of calculating fee-for-service benefits is the usual, customary, and reasonable concept. Usual refers to the fee that the doctor charges private patients for a specific service. Customary fees are established if the fees fall in the same range of fees of several doctors within the same geographic area. Customary fees between specialists are grouped together and are considered separately from the general practitioners' fees. Reasonable is the concept applied to justify higher fees in cases when treatment rendered required extra time or skill due to the nature of the procedure. In these special circumstances, the doctor will increase the usual fee.

60. (A) When storing supplies, frequently used items should be stored where they can be reached easily. The operatory or dental laboratory storage areas are best suited for small consumable items and supplies that are used continuously. Manufacturers' storage recommendations must be considered when storing supplies. X-ray film should not be stored near a light or heat source, and certain types of cements must be stored at room temperature. Less frequently used supplies should be stored in a supply room and need not be as easily accessible.

61. (D)

62. (C)

63. (A)

64. (B)

65. (E)

66. (D) The patient account record, or ledger card, is used by the business assistant to record all financial transactions, including payments, charges, credits, and current balance information. Necessary information includes patient's home address and telephone number, work number and work address, and insurance information. The number of hours worked per week is not indicated as necessary information on a patient account record.

67. (D) A treatment plan is a systematic approach to accomplishing the dental needs of the patient. This plan is made after evaluating the diagnostic materials gathered from and about the patient (e.g., medical and dental histories, radiographs, study models, clinical examination). Elements of a treatment plan include the procedure, the priority of the procedure, who will perform the task, and the amount of time the procedure requires.

68. (A) A running inventory is a system of altering the supply list to know what is present in the office. This list is updated continuously as the supplies are used. This type of system is especially important for disposable supplies.

69. (B) The advantage of purchasing a large quantity of a particular supply at one time is to save money. The drawbacks are the storage space needed and the shelf life of the material, which might expire before the material is used.

70. (D) When recalling patients by telephone, the business assistant should have the patient's recall record ready for reference.

71. (A) All account transactions should be entered promptly on the daily journal page and the patient ledger card. The patient ledger card keeps an ongoing record of all charges, payments, insurance reimbursements, and outstanding balance information that may be necessary for collections. Charge slips are written forms of interoffice communication relating information about the current account balance and the fees charged for the services performed at that visit.

72. (C) An office manual is most effective when it is organized by the dentist and the staff in keeping with the office's philosophy, goals, and objectives.

73. (D) Pegboard accounting materials do not include bank deposit slips. The bank deposit slip keeps an itemized record of all the checks and cash payments. The deposit slip must contain the doctor's name, business address, and bank account number. After completion of the deposit slip, the money is ready to be deposited in the bank. A record of the deposit is recorded in the office account ledger.

74. (D) If the dental treatment has been completed and the account fully paid, the file is no longer considered active.

75. (A) The total fee for his dental treatment is $85.

76. (B) Money received in the dental practice must be placed in the bank. A deposit slip furnished by the bank is completed daily, detailing all of the checks and currency collected for that day. Checks and currency are listed separately on a deposit slip. Entries must be made in ink, legibly, and in duplicate (carbon copy). The patient's account record must be adjusted to reflect the amount of the check written to the dental practice before depositing. Checks do not need to be listed in alphabetical order but must be endorsed properly in order to be deposited.

77. **(C)** A returned check (a check that has bounced) must be charged back against the patient's account and subtracted from the office income bank balance. Allow the patient to clear the outstanding balance before proceeding with other dental treatment.

78. **(A)** A stop payment order on a check may be requested if there is reason to believe that a check has been lost. Payment can be stopped by filling out proper forms provided directly at the bank or by a telephone request to the bank. A stop payment order does not indicate insufficient funds.

79. **(A)** Daily proof-of-posting serves to double check all entries and transactions made on the daily journal page. This system requires that each of the columns must be totaled and balanced to ensure accuracy. The cash drawer also must balance with the received on accounts entries. If daily record keeping procedures are handled by a computer system, the columns can be totaled automatically.

80. **(B)**

81. **(C)**

82. **(B)**

83. **(C)**

84. **(D)**

85. **(B)**

86. **(D)** The office manual does not include payroll records. Every office should have an office manual that is updated periodically to accommodate changes in office procedures and policies. The office manual may also serve as a procedural guide for training new staff members. Medical emergency procedures and the goals and objectives of the dental practice also are defined in the office manual.

87. **(D)** When a patient is injured by a dentist's employee, both the employee and the dentist are liable. Under the principle of respondeat superior, the dentist is automatically associated and brought into the legal suit with the employee.

88. **(C)** Using eye contact during an employment interview is important and a necessary part of effective communication. Immediately discussing salary and hours is not recommended at the start of an interview, but these are issues that do need to be addressed at some point during the interview. A professional appearance is required for employment success.

89. **(D)** Consent to an operation or to a course of treatment may be expressed or implied. A patient may approve of dental treatment by formally giving written consent by placing his or her signature on office consent forms or treatment plan forms. Implied consent is not as clearly defined but is interpreted by a patient's actions and behavior. When a patient offers to open his or her mouth for an examination, he or she is agreeing to treatment.

90. **(C)** Anything done to a person without his or her consent is termed a trespass. A trespass action may be interpreted by law as "an unconsented touching." The importance of obtaining patient consent either through an expressed contract (in writing) or an implied contract (mutual agreement by 2 persons) before rendering dental treatment is necessary to avoid possible charges of trespass.

91. **(C)** The most important piece of evidence used by the defense in most malpractice cases is the patient dental record. All patient dental records must be well documented and filled out in ink. Radiographs, laboratory reports, and study models also are part of the permanent dental record and must be correctly labeled. All entries should be dated and followed by a detailed description of each procedure performed. The initials or complete last name of the ancillary staff performing direct patient care should follow the dental entry. Medical health history questionnaires should be updated periodically and initialed by the reviewer.

92. **(C)** Professional liability claims are most likely to be based on the charge of faulty or erroneous diagnosis, based on the principle that the doctor's reasonable and prudent diagnosis determines the type and extent of dental treatment rendered to the patient. Every patient can expect the right to a reasonable standard of skill and care when seeking dental treatment. If this right is abused or neglected, a malpractice suit may be initiated.

93. (D) Negligence may be defined as the failure to exercise reasonable and ordinary care to avoid injury to another. In health care settings, the charge of negligence or lack of reasonable care in serving a patient by the health professional is termed malpractice.

94. (D) Receivables refer to money outstanding for treatment completed.

95. (A) Open accounts are the most difficult ones to collect, since statements on open accounts usually are sent to patients after treatment has been rendered. This gives patients the option of paying at their convenience, which can increase the office's accounts receivable status.

96. (D) Canceled checks are checks that have been paid and charged to the depositor's account. On receipt of the office bank statement, the canceled checks should be reviewed and verified against the office checkbook and bank statement. A record of all canceled checks should be kept on file for future reference, or the information should be stored in a computer system.

97. (A) Petty cash is a small amount of cash kept in the office to purchase miscellaneous inexpensive items for the office (e.g., postage stamps, erasers). The business assistant may keep the petty cash vouchers, and all transactions should be dated and recorded. The petty cash fund is determined and replenished according to the doctor's and office's needs.

98. (B) A cashier's check is drawn by a bank on its own funds in exchange for an individual's personal check or cash. Cashier's checks must be endorsed by the recipient.

99. (D) Bank service charges have been subtracted previously from the bank statement total by the banking organization; this is not a step in reconciling a bank statement. Balancing (reconciling) the checkbook promptly against the bank statement is an important procedure and includes calculations involving outstanding checks, deposits in transit, and cross-checking canceled checks against the bank statement. All canceled checks and bank statements should be stored for future reference.

100. **(C)**   The business assistant may often be involved in the initial or preliminary interview process and the supervision and training of new staff members in office policies and procedures.

101. **(D)**   On occasion, a disruptive patient or patients who present unusual behavior in the patient waiting room may require a firm direct approach. The assistant must always handle this type of situation in a professional manner. Patients suspected of substance abuse or disruptive patients who present irrational behavior should be rescheduled.

102. **(C)**   Appointment control will prevent overcrowding, keep hours within desired limits, organize the dentist's production time, assign tasks to the proper individual, and provide patients with definite appointment information.

103. **(A)**   Important reasons for record keeping are that it legally avoids possible malpractice involvement, provides an accurate history of treatment success and failure, provides production records, enables others to carry on treatment, and allows future treatment to be based on past performance, such as reaction to anesthesia and payment.

104. **(B)**   During an office medical emergency situation the business assistant should assist the doctor and chairside assistant where needed and call for medical emergency support services if indicated. Each member of the office staff should be trained in medical emergency protocol.

Comprehensive Simulated Exam

DIRECTIONS: Each of the questions or incomplete statements in this section is followed by four suggested answers or completions. Select the **ONE** lettered answer or completion that is **BEST** in each case.

1. Health history questionnaires must be completed
   - **A.** at every dental appointment
   - **B.** before rendering clinical dental care
   - **C.** in ink at the end of the dental treatment
   - **D.** only if a surgical procedure is indicated

2. A common drug used in the dental office to decrease anxiety is
   - **A.** nitrous oxide
   - **B.** caffeine
   - **C.** aspirin
   - **D.** benzocaine

3. Protective barriers are necessary when
   - **A.** confirming appointments
   - **B.** presenting toothbrush instruction
   - **C.** ordering supplies
   - **D.** sterilizing instruments

4. The main role of the assistant in preventive dentistry is
   A. dispensing fluoride rinses
   B. taking x-rays
   C. patient education
   D. recording vital signs

5. If caries is present on the lingual pit of tooth No. 7, it is classified as
   A. Class V
   B. Class IV
   C. Class I
   D. Class III

6. Which of the following is **NOT** used to evaluate an amalgam restoration?
   A. Mirror
   B. Burnisher
   C. Articulating paper
   D. Dental floss

7. Which of the following pieces of equipment should be disinfected after treatment of each patient?
   A. Handpieces
   B. Curettes
   C. Film holders
   D. Light handles

8. Instruments used on a patient with a history of hepatitis B should be sterilized by
   A. scrubbing with alcohol
   B. heating in a dry oven for 20 min.
   C. a cold disinfectant method
   D. a steam sterilization (autoclave) method

9. A dental assistant may expose radiographs if
   A. the dentist gives permission
   B. he or she is a certified dental assistant
   C. it is permissible in the state in which he or she is employed
   D. he or she is supervised by the dentist or hygienist

10. The amount of radiation a person receives
    A. begins anew each day
    B. is cumulative only on the skin
    C. is cumulative in the entire body
    D. is not harmful in small doses

11. A technique used to measure the operator's exposure to radiation is
    A. to check the color of the operator's fingernails
    B. for the operator to wear a radiation film badge
    C. to multiply the number of films the operator has exposed by 0.1 rem
    D. to count the number of full mouth x-ray series taken

12. Accumulated radiation dosage for those who work with radiation may not exceed
    A. 0.1 rem/wk
    B. 1 rem/wk
    C. 10 rem/wk
    D. 100 rem/wk

13. To avoid exposure to secondary radiation, the operator should stand
    A. at least 6′ from the x-ray head
    B. 2′ to the right of the primary beam
    C. any distance in back of the x-ray head
    D. 4′ in front of the patient

14. The most effective way to reduce gonadal exposure from x-rays is to
    A. increase the kVp
    B. use a leaded lap apron
    C. increase vertical angulation
    D. use ultraspeed film

15. After each use, the leaded lap apron must be
    A. stored in the darkroom
    B. folded neatly and stored in the operatory
    C. draped over a support rod unfolded
    D. discarded for appropriate infection control

16. The best technique for reducing the radiation exposure to both patient and operator is the use of
   A. an automatic timer
   B. fast film
   C. thinner films
   D. a thicker cellulose acetate base

17. If a caustic chemical comes in contact with the eyes, which of the following steps must be taken?
   A. Close eyes and apply a wet compress to forehead
   B. Flush eyes with water and seek medical attention as quickly as possible
   C. Close eyes and apply dark tinted safety glasses
   D. An incident report documenting route of exposure must be made

18. Labeling of hazardous products in the dental office is required if the hazardous product
   A. is to be used immediately within an 8-hr. shift
   B. has an original label from the manufacturer
   C. is a prescription item
   D. is transferred to a secondary container

19. OSHA guidelines require employers to establish a written exposure control plan that includes
   A. engineering and work practice controls
   B. identification of job classifications and risks
   C. information on exposure incident reporting
   D. employee's medical records

20. The best way to recap a needle is to
   A. utilize the one-handed scoop technique
   B. disengage the needle from syringe, then recap
   C. use a puncture-proof sharps container
   D. have the dentist replace the cap using the two-handed technique

21. Following OSHA guidelines if an employee refuses to obtain the hepatitis vaccination, the employer is required to
   A. dismiss the employee
   B. ask the employee not to participate in surgical procedures
   C. have the employee sign an informed refusal/declination form
   D. have the employee double glove for all procedures

22. OSHA standards regarding contaminated laundry include all of the following **EXCEPT**
   A. it must be handled as little as possible
   B. laundry transport bags must be labeled with a biohazard symbol
   C. a washer and dryer may be used on-site
   D. employee training is not required

23. Orthodontics is the dental specialty that deals with the
   A. diseases and abnormal conditions of the hard and soft tissues of the oral cavity
   B. treatment of pulpal and periapical diseases of the teeth
   C. growth and development of the jaws and face
   D. prevention and education of dental health problems on a community level

24. The condition in which the mandible is located ahead of the maxilla is called
   A. prognathism
   B. micrognathism
   C. retrusion
   D. centric relation

25. The best way to motivate adolescents to practice good oral hygiene habits is by
   A. establishing feelings of security
   B. relating it to social acceptance and appearance
   C. explaining monetary considerations
   D. providing a detailed explanation of dental plaque

26. A headgear appliance is worn
   A. during active play and while sleeping
   B. as the orthodontist prescribes
   C. a minimum of 8 hr. a day, 5 days a week
   D. 24 hr. a day except while eating

27. A positioner is worn
   A. in place of a fixed appliance
   B. for gross tooth movement
   C. to separate the teeth before banding
   D. after the removal of fixed appliances

28. Cephalometry is
   A. taking measurements of the skull
   B. compression of the skull
   C. the study of the soft tissues of the head
   D. a technique for maintaining orthodontic movement

29. An "open bite" refers to a condition wherein
   A. there are no posterior teeth
   B. there are spaces between teeth in the same arch
   C. the anterior teeth do not contact
   D. the teeth contact only during mastication

30. Overjet is the
   A. horizontal distance between maxillary and mandibular teeth
   B. coronal length of maxillary anterior teeth
   C. vertical overlap of maxillary and mandibular anterior teeth
   D. labioversion of the mandibular teeth

31. A biopsy is
   A. any lesion in the oral cavity
   B. the surgical removal of an abscessed tooth
   C. the removal of tissue for diagnostic purposes
   D. the radical removal of a cancerous lesion

32. An instrument that holds a tissue flap away from the operating field is called a
- **A.** pick
- **B.** retractor
- **C.** elevator
- **D.** hemostat

33. An impaction is
- **A.** a succedaneous tooth
- **B.** a tooth that will not erupt fully
- **C.** any tooth that is ankylosed
- **D.** a supernumerary tooth

34. General anesthetics are administered
- **A.** for nerve blocks
- **B.** routinely in most dental offices
- **C.** to render the patient unconscious
- **D.** without any risks

35. Before assisting in surgery in the hospital operating room, the assistant should perform a thorough surgical scrub for approximately
- **A.** 1 min.
- **B.** 3 min.
- **C.** 5 min.
- **D.** 10 min.

36. The three body systems that are monitored on a patient during general anesthesia or intravenous sedation are the
- **A.** cardiovascular, lymphatic, and peripheral systems
- **B.** cardiovascular, central venous, and muscular systems
- **C.** cardiovascular, central nervous, and respiratory systems
- **D.** digestive, respiratory, and lymphatic systems

37. When palpating the pulse, you should be aware of the
- **A.** location, placement, and strength of the pulse
- **B.** rate, rhythm, and strength of the pulse
- **C.** respiration rate per minute
- **D.** patient's body temperature

38. Dental implants are classified in which set of three categories?
   A. Endosteal, periosteal, and transosteal
   B. Subperiosteal, transosteal, and subendosteal
   C. Endosteal, subperiosteal, and transosteal
   D. Subperiosteal, endosteal, and subtransosteal

39. The condition in which a patient lacks oxygen is called
   A. hyperventilation
   B. hypoxia
   C. anoxia
   D. syncope

40. The patient's clinical record must include
   A. laboratory invoices
   B. medical health questionnaire
   C. study models
   D. insurance forms

41. The assistant holds the hand instrument to be transferred between the
   A. thumb and forefinger
   B. small finger and palm
   C. thumb and palm
   D. small finger and forefinger

42. During the administration of local anesthesia, aspiration will
   A. damage the mandibular artery
   B. be extremely painful
   C. determine if the lumen of the needle is in a blood vessel
   D. ensure profound anesthesia

43. When working in the anterior part of the mouth, the high-volume evacuation tip is held
   A. below the incisal edge of the tooth being prepared
   B. on the opposite side of the tooth being prepared
   C. in the retromolar area
   D. in the vestibule

44. Angle's classification of malocclusion is based on the
A. shape of the maxilla
B. relationship between the first molars and the orbit of the eye
C. relationship between the maxillary and mandibular first molars
D. number of teeth in the mandible

45. The normal reading for blood pressure is
A. 120/80
B. 140/100
C. 160/80
D. 180/60

46. To increase the penetrating quality of an x-ray beam, the auxiliary must
A. increase kVp
B. decrease kVp
C. increase mA
D. increase FFD

47. A test for quality control relative to manual processing may be accomplished utilizing a
A. test tube
B. darkroom safelight
C. water thermometer
D. stepwedge

48. The dental assistant must utilize which of the following personal protective equipment (PPE) when exposing films?
A. Safety goggles
B. Gloves
C. Chin-length face shield
D. Tinted lenses

49. The raised button on the radiograph aids in
A. determining film speed
B. processing
C. drying
D. mounting

50. The purpose of the lead foil in dental film is to
    A. provide stiffness to the film
    B. reduce film fogging
    C. absorb the primary beam
    D. prevent scattered radiation to the patient

51. The detection of interproximal caries is seen best with a (an)
    A. occlusal film
    B. panorex film
    C. bite-wing film
    D. lateral head plate

52. The best place to store unexposed x-ray film is in a
    A. lead container
    B. puncture-resistant sealed container
    C. darkroom
    D. warm area protected from stray radiation

53. The periapical film reveals
    A. the entire jaw
    B. upper and lower teeth in the same film
    C. interproximal caries
    D. the entire tooth, including the apex

54. A material or substance that does **NOT** stop or absorb x-rays is known as
    A. radiographic
    B. radiopaque
    C. radiolucent
    D. radiodontic

55. A material or substance that stops or absorbs x-rays is known as
    A. radiographic
    B. radiopaque
    C. radiolucent
    D. radiodontic

56. What is the small circular radiolucency near the roots of the mandibular premolars called?
   A. Lingual foramen
   B. Mental foramen
   C. Mandibular foramen
   D. Incisive foramen

57. What is the thin radiopaque band between the maxillary incisors called?
   A. Median palatine suture
   B. Nasal septum
   C. Inverted Y
   D. Zygoma

58. Which of these appears radiolucent?
   A. Caries
   B. Calculus
   C. Torus
   D. Root tips

59. What is the large radiolucent area shown on maxillary molar radiographs called?
   A. Maxillary sinus
   B. Maxillary septum
   C. Maxillary tuberosity
   D. Maxillary sequestrum

60. The ala-tragus line is parallel to the floor when taking
   A. mandibular occlusal films
   B. mandibular periapical films
   C. extraoral films only
   D. maxillary periapical films

61. "Ethics" refers to
   A. accreditation by the ADA
   B. professional standards of conduct
   C. jurisprudence
   D. membership in the ADAA

62. What determines which duties the dental assistant can perform?
   A. State law
   B. Federal law
   C. Common law
   D. The dentist

63. The period of time in which a patient may bring suit against a dentist is known as
   A. probationary time
   B. libel
   C. tort
   D. statute of limitations

64. A patient suing for malpractice may include in the suit
   A. the dental assistant
   B. the dentist only
   C. the hygienist and dentist only
   D. anyone working in the dental practice

65. Patient records are
   A. public information
   B. available only to relatives
   C. confidential records and private property
   D. released at the assistant's discretion

66. An appropriate response when answering the phone is
   A. "This is Dr. Smith's office. Chris Jones speaking. May I help you?"
   B. "Who's calling?"
   C. "With whom would you like to speak?"
   D. "May I help you?"

67. A patient calls and complains about the treatment given. The receptionist should
   A. justify the dentist's position
   B. engage in a verbal duel
   C. take the patient's side
   D. allow the dentist to handle the situation

68. A case presentation is a
  A. treatment conference with the patient
  B. case that is sent to the laboratory for construction
  C. paper or speech presented by the doctor to a dental society
  D. study model used to diagnose a case

69. Which person traditionally controls the appointment book?
  A. Dentist
  B. Chairside assistant
  C. Receptionist
  D. Hygienist

70. Overhead is
  A. net income
  B. the cost necessary to practice dentistry
  C. assets of the practice
  D. the break-even production point

71. Under the OSHA (Occupational Safety Health Administration) standard, the records of an employee's exposure incident are to be
  A. entered into the office computer data bank for easy access
  B. kept confidential and filed in the employee's medical record
  C. faxed to the employee's private physician
  D. kept on file for 1 full year

72. When generating and processing electronic insurance claims through the office computer system it is necessary to
  A. log the information into the daily appointment schedule
  B. enter the information onto a deposit slip
  C. keep a backup file and paper record of claim
  D. mail a copy to the insurance company

73. A day sheet in each treatment room provides which of the following data?
  A. Any serious medical problem that could affect treatment
  B. The patient's occupation
  C. The procedure to be performed and length of the appointment
  D. The number of visits needed to complete treatment

74. An invoice is a
   A. statement of money collected
   B. bill for items shipped
   C. cash receipt
   D. form of vertical filing

75. Mr. Jones completed his dental treatment in September. For a 6-month recall he should return in
   A. January
   B. March
   C. April
   D. June

76. The color of the oxygen cylinder tank is always
   A. green
   B. blue
   C. red
   D. white

77. Proper preparation of a victim for artificial respiration is
   A. wipe foreign matter from mouth and tilt head backward with chin pointing downward
   B. wipe foreign matter from mouth and tilt head backward with chin pointing upward
   C. tilt head backward with chin pointing upward, put one hand under victim's neck, and lift
   D. do not wipe foreign matter from mouth but lift victim's neck to raise chin

78. When having an alginate impression of the upper arch taken, the patient should be seated in a (an)
   A. slightly reclined position with the chin tilted downward
   B. upright position with head tilted forward
   C. upright position with head tilted back
   D. supine position

79. A Tofflemire matrix prepared for tooth No. 28 can also be used on teeth in which other quadrant?
 A. Maxillary left
 B. Mandibular right
 C. Maxillary right
 D. Mandibular left

80. What instruments are best suited for removing excess cement from the teeth?
 A. Spatula and scalpel
 B. Dull chisel and mallet
 C. Ball burnisher and explorer
 D. Explorer and scaler

81. When working with a visible light cure unit
 A. the dental unit light must be set on low
 B. a face shield may be worn in place of a face mask
 C. protective visible light eyewear is required
 D. protective eyewear is not necessary

82. Light pressure should be used when polishing with a rubber cup so as not to cause the cup to
 A. flange into the gingival sulcus
 B. fray
 C. unscrew from the prophy angle
 D. cause any unnecessary frictional heat

83. The most common form of fluoride used with the rigid tray system is
 A. sodium fluoride (NaF)
 B. stannous fluoride paste
 C. liquid fluoride supplements
 D. acidulated phosphate fluoride gel

84. The Dental Practice Act
 A. is operated as an agency of the federal government
 B. is under the jurisdiction of the American Dental Association
 C. defines the practice and regulates dentistry in each state
 D. certifies dental assistants

85. When removing sutures, you must cut
A. anywhere, as long as you can get the suture out
B. in back of the knot and pull knot through tissue
C. just below the knot with suture scissors
D. the knot off, then remove suture gently with a hemostat

86. Glass ionomer cements may be used for
A. permanent restorations
B. luting procedures
C. insulating bases
D. sealants

87. When teaching toothbrushing, the emphasis should be on
A. brushing at least once a day
B. brushing three times a day
C. brushing before bedtime
D. complete removal of plaque regardless of brushing time

88. A mixed dentition consists of
A. deciduous and permanent teeth existing simultaneously in a child's mouth
B. deciduous teeth in the wrong places
C. permanent teeth that are rotated
D. permanent teeth in the wrong places

89. A "furcation" in periodontics refers to
A. a surgical procedure
B. the mobility of anterior teeth
C. the radicular area of multirooted teeth
D. a dry mouth

90. The function of the periodontium is to
A. prevent caries
B. support the teeth
C. prevent vertical food impaction
D. aid the tongue in cleansing the teeth

91. If you had an emergency in the office involving syncope, what would you be treating?
   A. Headache
   B. Hyperventilation
   C. Cardiac arrest
   D. Fainting

92. A patient having an angina attack suffers from which medical problem?
   A. Diabetes
   B. Heart trouble
   C. High blood pressure
   D. Fever

93. Which of the following is most descriptive of someone in shock?
   A. Face pale, pulse strong, breathing regular
   B. Nervousness, face flushed, pulse rapid
   C. Skin cool and clammy, pulse weak, breathing irregular
   D. Nausea, breathing rapid, pusle strong

94. Accounts receivable are
   A. monies owed to the dentist from insurance carriers
   B. all monies owed to the dentist for completed treatment
   C. all monies that the dentist owes to creditors
   D. all monies owed to the dentist for future treatment

95. Insurance codes and nomenclature for specific dental treatment procedures are obtained in the
   A. CDT published by the American Dental Association
   B. CDC (Centers for Disease Control) publication
   C. third-party carrier's manual
   D. office procedures manual

96. Federal regulations that affect the practice of dentistry regarding "public accommodations" include the
   A. Occupational Safety Health Administration (OSHA) regulations
   B. Environmental Protection Agency (EPA) regulations
   C. Internal Revenue Service (IRS) regulations
   D. Americans with Disabilities Act (ADA)-Title III regulations

97. Every dental office is required to maintain a written hazard communication program, which contains all of the following **EXCEPT**
   A. material safety data sheets (MSDS)
   B. laundry schedules and costs
   C. hazardous chemicals log
   D. employee training records for Hazard Communication Standard

98. Negligence is
   A. a legal duty to the public
   B. a general duty to the dental profession
   C. a general duty to the legal profession
   D. the failure to exercise reasonable and ordinary care to avoid injury to others

99. If an immunized dental health care worker experiences a percutaneous injury from a patient who is HBsAG (hepatitis B surface antigen) negative, the exposed worker should
   A. not need further treatment once immunized
   B. start the hepatitis vaccine series immediately
   C. test for antibody to hepatitis B surface antigen
   D. request HBIG (hepatitis B immune globulin) booster

100. The OSHA Hazard Communication Standard provides the employee with information regarding all of the following **EXCEPT**
   A. fire safety and clean-up procedures for acid spills
   B. ventilation requirements for chemical vapor sterilization
   C. training sessions for safe handling of hazardous chemicals including radiographic processing chemicals
   D. education regarding the benefits of vaccinations

Comprehensive Simulated Exam

Answer Key

1. B	26. B	51. C	76. A
2. A	27. D	52. A	77. D
3. D	28. A	53. D	78. B
4. C	29. C	54. C	79. A
5. C	30. A	55. B	80. D
6. B	31. C	56. B	81. C
7. D	32. B	57. B	82. D
8. D	33. B	58. A	83. D
9. C	34. C	59. A	84. C
10. C	35. D	60. D	85. C
11. B	36. C	61. B	86. A
12. A	37. B	62. A	87. D
13. A	38. C	63. D	88. A
14. B	39. B	64. D	89. C
15. C	40. B	65. C	90. B
16. B	41. A	66. A	91. D
17. C	42. C	67. D	92. B
18. D	43. B	68. A	93. C
19. A	44. C	69. C	94. B
20. A	45. A	70. B	95. A
21. C	46. A	71. B	96. D
22. D	47. D	72. C	97. B
23. C	48. B	73. C	98. D
24. A	49. D	74. B	99. A
25. B	50. B	75. B	100. D

Bibliography

American Dental Assistants Association Department of Continuing Education. *ICE PACK.* 1995.

American Heart Association. *A Student Handbook for Cardiopulmonary Resuscitation and First Aid for Choking.* 1993.

American National Red Cross. *American Red Cross Standard First Aid Workbook.* 1988.

American Red Cross. *Advanced First Aid and Emergency Care,* 2nd ed. New York: Doubleday and Co, Inc, 1980.

Anthony CP, Thibodeau GA. *Structure and Function of the Body,* 6th ed. St. Louis: CV Mosby Co, 1980.

Atchison KA. *Radiographic Safety.* Western Dental Education Center Correspondence Course. Los Angeles: Department of Veterans Affairs, West Los Angeles VA Medical Center, 1987.

Boucher CO. *Boucher's Clinical Dental Terminology: Glossary of Accepted Terms in All Disciplines of Dentistry,* 4th ed. St. Louis: CV Mosby Co, 1993.

Brown SK. *Infection Control in Dental Practices.* Miami, FL: Health Studies Institute, Inc, 1993.

Butsumyo D, Deboom G, Lynne S, Parrot K. *Principles and Practice of Dental Radiography.* Los Angeles: Western Dental Education Center Correspondence Course. Department of Veterans Affairs, West Los Angeles VA Medical Center, 1988.

Caplan CM. *Dental Practice Management Encyclopedia.* Penn Well, 1985.

Carter LM, Yaman P, Ladley BA, eds. *Dental Instruments.* St. Louis: CV Mosby Co, 1981.

261

Chasteen JE. *Essentials of Clinical Dentistry Assisting,* 4th ed. St. Louis: CV Mosby Co, 1989.

Chen PS. *Chemistry: Inorganic, Organic and Biological,* 2nd ed. New York: Harper & Row Publishers Inc, 1980.

Christensen GJ. Glass Ionomer as a Luting Material. *J Am Dent Assoc.* 1990; 120: 55–57.

Ciancio SG, Bourgault PC. *Clinical Pharmacology for Dental Professionals,* 3rd ed. Chicago: Year Book Medical Publishers, Inc, 1989.

Cochran DL, Klakwarf K, Brunsvold M. *Plaque and Calculus Removal Considerations for the Professional.* Chicago: Quintessence Publishing Co, Inc, 1994.

Cottone JA, Molinari JA, Terezhalmy G. *Practical Infection Control in Dentistry,* 2nd ed. Mavern, PA: Lea & Febiger, 1996.

Craig RG. *Restorative Dental Materials,* 9th ed. St Louis: CV Mosby Co, 1993.

Davis K. *Training Manual for Oral and Maxillofacial Surgery Assistants,* 3rd ed. Lomita, CA: King Printing, 1996.

deLyre WR, Johnson N. *Essentials of Dental Radiology for Dental Assistants and Hygienists,* 5th ed. Stamford, CT: Appleton & Lange, 1995.

Domer LR, Snyder TL, Heid DW, eds. *Dental Practice Management.* St. Louis: CV Mosby Co, 1980.

Eastman Kodak Company. *Successful Panoramic Radiography.* Rochester, NY, 1993.

Eastman Kodak Company. *Quality Assurance in Dental Radiography.* Rochester, NY, 1990.

Eastman Kodak Company. *Radiation Safety in Dental Radiography.* Rochester, NY, 1990.

Eastman Kodak Company. *X-rays in Dentistry.* Rochester, NY, 1977.

Ehrlich A. *Business Administration for the Dental Assistant,* 4th ed. Champaign, IL: Colwell Systems, 1991.

Ehrlich A. *Nutrition and Dental Health.* Albany, NY: Delmar Publications, 1987.

Facts About AIDS for the Dental Team, 2nd ed. American Dental Association Council on Dental Therapeutics, Chicago: American Dental Association, October 1988.

Finkbeiner BL, Johnson CS. *Comprehensive Dental Assisting.* St. Louis: CV Mosby Co, 1994.

Finkbeiner BL, Patt JC. *Practice Management for the Dental Team,* 3rd ed. St. Louis: CV Mosby Co, 1991.

Frommer HH. *Radiology for Dental Auxiliaries,* 5th ed. St. Louis: CV Mosby Co, 1992.

Fuller JL, Denehy GE. *Concise Dental Anatomy and Morphology,* 2nd ed. Chicago: Year Book Medical Publishers, Inc, 1984.

Gilmore, HW, et al. *Operative Dentistry,* 4th ed. St. Louis: CV Mosby Co, 1982.

Giunta JL. *Oral Pathology,* 3rd ed. Philadelphia: BC Decker, Inc, 1989.

Goss CM. *Gray's Anatomy,* 30th ed. Philadelphia: Lea & Febiger Publishers, 1985.

Goth A. *Medical Pharmacology,* 10th ed. St. Louis: CV Mosby Co, 1981.

Guthrie HA. *Human Nutrition.* St. Louis: CV Mosby Co, 1994.

Harris NO, Christen AG. *Primary Preventive Dentistry,* 4th ed. Stamford, CT: Appleton & Lange, 1994.

Hefferson JJ, Ayer WA, Koehler HM, eds. *Foods, Nutrition and Dental Health,* Vol. I. South, IL: Pathodox Publishers, 1980.

Hooley J, Whitacre R. *Medications Used in Oral Surgery,* 3rd ed. Seattle: Stoma Press, Inc, 1984.

Infection Control in the Dental Environment. Department of Veterans Affairs, American Dental Association, Department of Health and Human Services and Centers for Disease Control. Washington, DC: Eastern Dental Education Center Learning Resources Center, Veterans Administration, 1989.

Jawetz E, et al. *Review of Medical Microbiology,* 20th ed. Stamford, CT: Appleton & Lange, 1995.

Keeton WT. *Biological Science,* 3rd ed. New York: WW Norton and Co, 1980.

Kumar, Angell M. *Basic Pathology,* 5th ed. Philadelphia: WB Saunders Co, 1992.

Ladley BA, Wilson SA. *Review of Dental Assisting.* St. Louis: CV Mosby Co, 1980.

Langland OE. *Radiography for Dental Hygienists & Dental Assistants,* 3rd ed. Springfield, IL: Charles C Thomas Publishers, 1988.

Little JW, Falace DA. *Dental Management of the Medically Compromised Patient,* 4th ed. St. Louis: CV Mosby Co, 1993.

Malamed SF. *Handbook of Medical Emergencies in the Dental Office,* 4th ed. St. Louis: CV Mosby Co, 1993.

Manson-Hing LR. *Fundamentals of Dental Radiography,* 3rd ed. Philadelphia: Lea & Febiger Publishers, 1990.

Miles D, Van Dis M, Jensen C, Ferretti A. *Radiographic Imaging for Dental Auxiliaries,* 2nd ed. Philadelphia: WB Saunders Co, 1993.

Miller BF, Keane CB. *Encyclopedia and Dictionary of Medicine, Nursing, and Allied Health,* 4th ed. Philadelphia: WB Saunders Co, 1987.

Miller CH, Palenik CJ. *Infection Control and Management of Hazardous Materials for the Dental Team.* St. Louis: CV Mosby Co, 1994.

Miller F. *College Physics,* 6th ed. New York: Harcourt Brace Jovanovich, Inc, 1987.

Muma RD, Lyons B, Borucki MJ, Pollard RB. *HIV Manual for Health Care Professionals.* Stamford, CT: Appleton & Lange, 1994.

Newman HN. *Dental Plaque.* Springfield, IL: Charles C Thomas Publishers, 1980.

Olson S. *Dental Radiography Laboratory Manual.* Philadelphia: WB Saunders Co, 1995.

Orban B. *Oral History and Embryology,* 9th ed. St. Louis: CV Mosby Co, 1980.

Peterson LJ. *Contemporary Oral and Maxillofacial Surgery,* 2nd ed. St. Louis: CV Mosby Co, 1993.

Philips RN. *Elements of Dental Materials for Dental Hygienists and Assistants,* 5th ed. Philadelphia: WB Saunders Co, 1994.

Randolph PM, Dennison CI. *Diet, Nutrition, and Dentistry.* St. Louis: CV Mosby Co, 1981.

Richardson RE, Barton RE. *The Dental Assistant,* 6th ed. New York: McGraw-Hill Inc, 1988.

Rose LF, Kaye D. *Internal Medicine for Dentistry,* 2nd ed. St. Louis: CV Mosby Co, 1990.

Rowe AHR, Alexander AG. *Clinical Methods, Medicine, Pathology and Pharmacology—A Companion to Dental Studies,* Vol 2. Boston: Blackwell Scientific Publications, 1988.

Sande MA, Volberding PA. *The Medical Management of AIDS,* 4th ed. Philadelphia: WB Saunders Co, 1994.

Schwarzrock SP, Jensen JR. *Effective Dental Assisting,* 7th ed. Dubuque, IA: William C Brown Co, 1991.

Section on Instructional System Design, Department of Pediodontology, School of Dentistry, University of California, San Francisco. Plaque Control Instruction. Berkeley, CA: Praxis Publishing Co, 1978.

Seymour RA, Walton JG. *Adverse Drug Reactions in Dentistry.* New York: Oxford University Press, 1989.

Shafer WG, Hine MK, Levy BM. *Textbook of Oral Pathology,* 4th ed. Philadelphia: WB Saunders Co, 1983.

Shin D, Avers J. *AIDS/HIV Reference Guide for Medical Professionals.* West Los Angeles, CA: CIRID/UCLA School of Medicine Publishers, 1988.

Sicher H. *Sicher's Oral Anatomy,* 8th ed. St. Louis: CV Mosby Co, 1988.

Skinner EW, Philips RW. *Skinner's Science of Dental Materials,* 9th ed. Philadelphia: WB Saunders Co, 1991.

Smith DC. Dental Cements. *Adv Dent Res.* 1988; 2:134–141.

Spohn EE, Halouski WA, Berry TC. *Operative Dentistry Procedures for Dental Auxiliaries.* St. Louis: CV Mosby Co, 1981.

Supplement—Handling Hazardous Chemicals General Guidelines, American Dental Association, 1995.

Suzuki M, Jordan R. Glass Ionomer—Composite Sandwich Technique. *J Am Dent Assoc.*1990; 120:55–57.

Thibodeau GA. *Anatomy and Physiology,* 3rd ed. St. Louis: CV Mosby Co, 1995.

Torres H, Ehrlich A, Bird D, Dietz E. *Modern Dental Assisting,* 5th ed. Philadelphia: WB Saunders Co, 1995.

Tyldesley WR. *Oral Medicine,* 3rd ed. New York: Oxford University Press, 1990.

U.S. Department of Labor, Office of Health Compliance Assistance. OSHA Hazard Communication Standard, *Code of Federal Regulations, #29,* Part 1910 et al, Feburary 9, 1994.

U.S. Department of Labor, Occupational Safety and Health Administration. *Controlling Occupational Exposure to Bloodborne Pathogens in Dentistry.* OSHA Publication 3129, 1992.

U.S. Department of Labor, Occupational Safety and Health Administration. *Chemical Hazard Communication.* OSHA Publication 3084 (Revised), 1988.

U.S. Department of Labor, Occupational Safety and Health Administration. *Hazard Communication Guidelines for Compliance.* OSHA Publication 3111, 1988.

Veterans Administration Medical Center. *Periodontal Resident Manual.* West Los Angeles, CA: VA Medical Center, 1990.

Wheeler S. *Dental Anatomy, Physiology and Occlusion,* 7th ed. Philadelphia: WB Saunders Co, 1992.

Wheeler S. *An Atlas of Tooth Form,* 5th ed. Philadelphia: WB Saunders Co, 1984.

Wilkins EM. *Clinical Practice of the Dental Hygienist,* 7th ed. Philadelphia: Lea & Febiger, 1994.

Woodall IR. *Legal, Ethical, and Management Aspects of the Dental Care System,* 3rd ed. St. Louis: CV Mosby Co, 1987.

Wuehrmann A, Manson-Hing LR. *Dental Radiology,* 5th ed. St. Louis: CV Mosby Co, 1981.

Zwemer TJ. *Boucher's Clinical Dental Terminology,* 4th ed. St. Louis: CV Mosby Co, 1993.

2. Hard Disk Installation from File Manager in Windows® 3.1 or 3.11

   a. Once the computer is started, insert the the MICROSTUDY disk marked INSTALL into the appropriate floppy drive.

   b. From File Manager, click on the floppy drive symbol where the MICROSTUDY INSTALL disk was inserted. Find the program file INSTALL.EXE and double on it to start the installation.

   c. INSTALL copies all required files from the designated floppy drive to the designated hard drive and its sub-directories, then creates a MICROSTUDY icon within a MICROSTUDY program group.

   d. Start MICROSTUDY by double clicking with a mouse on the MICROSTUDY program icon in the MICRO-STUDY group.

3. Hard Disk Installation from Start in Windows® 95

   a. Once the computer is started, insert the MICROSTUDY disk marked INSTALL into the appropriate floppy drive.

   b. Select Run from the Start Menu. Type **A:\INSTALL** or **B:\INSTALL** in the Command Line of Run, then press OK.

   c. INSTALL copies all required files from the designated floppy drive to the designated hard drive and its sub-directories, then creates a MICROSTUDY icon within a MICROSTUDY program group.

   d. Start MICROSTUDY by double clicking with a mouse on the MICROSTUDY program icon in the MICRO-STUDY group.

4. Hard Disk Installation from Explorer in Windows® 95

   a. Once the computer is started, insert the MICROSTUDY disk marked INSTALL into the appropriate floppy drive.

   b. From Explorer, click on the floppy drive symbol in which the MICROSTUDY INSTALL disk was inserted. Find the program file INSTALL.EXE and double click on it to start installation.

   c. INSTALL copies all required files from the designated floppy drive to the designated hard drive and its sub-directories, then creates a MICROSTUDY icon within a MICROSTUDY group.

   d. Start MICROSTUDY by double clicking with a mouse on the MICROSTUDY program icon in the MICRO-STUDY group.

Directions for Installing
MICROSTUDY®

MICROSTUDY® V3.1 FOR WINDOWS FEATURES

1. Quizzes consisting of chapter questions may be taken in the authors' original order or in a randomly scrambled order.

2. Follow-up tests are composed of missed-questions.

3. Electronic notebook enables students' comments to be entered and saved while studying, then recalled later for review, modifying or printing.

4. Customized comprehensive exams may be automatically built. These exams may be presented under NAPLEX simulation or in the standard MICROSTUDY simulated exam format.

5. Performance is monitored and a report card is assembled after each work session. Comprehensive exam statistics are tabulated and displayed for exam performance comparisons.

6. Digital timer shows elapsed study time.

7. Audio feedback that signals responses may be used.

8. A four-function memory calculator is available while studying.

MICROSTUDY® V3.1 FOR WINDOWS®
INSTALLATION AND STARTUP

1. Hard Disk Installation from Run in Windows® 3.1 or 3.11

   a. Once the computer is started, insert the MICROSTUDY disk marked INSTALL into the appropriate floppy drive.

   b. Select Run from under the File Menu. Type A:\INSTALL or B:\INSTALL in the Command Line of Run, then press OK.

   c. INSTALL copies all required files from the designated floppy drive to the designated hard drive and its subdirectories, then creates a MICROSTUDY icon within a MICROSTUDY program group.

   d. Start MICROSTUDY by double clicking with a mouse on the MICROSTUDY program icon in the MICROSTUDY group.